THE HOLISTIC HOME

FENG SHUI FOR MIND, BODY, SPIRIT, SPACE

LAURA BENKO

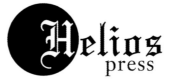

Helios press

Helios Press books may be purchased in bulk at special discounts for sales promotion, corporate gifts, fund-raising, or educational purposes. Special editions can also be created to specifications. For details, contact the Special Sales Department, Skyhorse Publishing, 307 West 36th Street, 11th Floor, New York, NY 10018 or info@skyhorsepublishing.com.

Helios® and Helios Press® are registered trademarks of Skyhorse Publishing, Inc.®, a Delaware corporation.

Visit our website at www.skyhorsepublishing.com.

10 9 8 7 6 5 4 3

Library of Congress Cataloging-in-Publication Data is available on file.

Cover design by Brian Peterson
Cover photo credit Susan Fisher Photography/Architecture, Interiors & Design
Haute Architecture DPC Diana Viñoly Interiors

Print ISBN: 978-1-63450-234-4
Ebook ISBN: 978-1-5107-0183-0

Printed in China

This book is dedicated to my mom and dad:

Barbara and Gene Benko, your endless support, unconditional love, and eternal optimism enabled me to achieve things I sometimes didn't think I could. Thank you for always believing in me. I love you more.

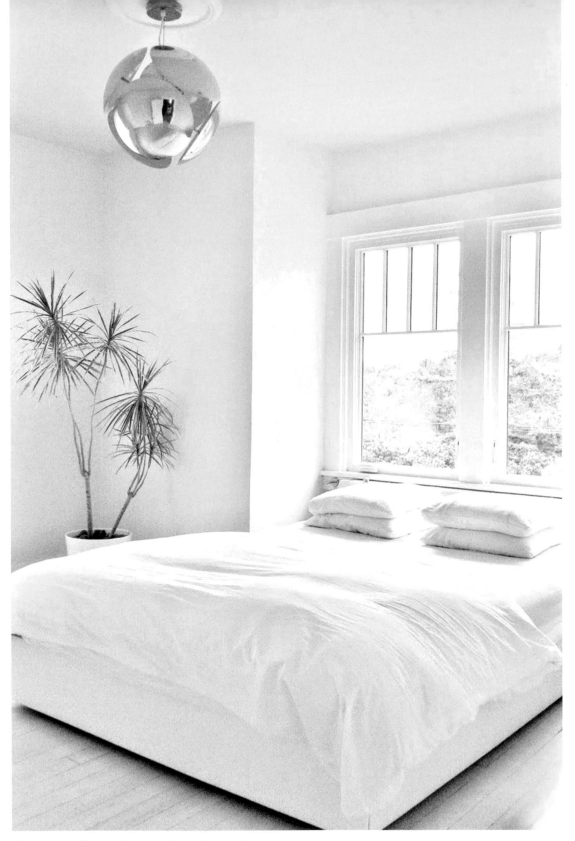

Courtesy of Bea Johnson, Zero Waste Home

Contents

CHAPTER ONE:
When Life Hits You On the Head, Listen   1

CHAPTER TWO:
Starting Clean: De-cluttering Your Mind, Body, and Spirit   14

CHAPTER THREE:
Get in Your Groove: Taking Cues from Nature   56

CHAPTER FOUR:
Go Deeper: Subconscious Symbolism in Your Home   83

CHAPTER FIVE:
Get In Position! Rule the World from Where You Sit,
Stand, and Sleep   109

CHAPTER SIX:
Yin and Yang: Finding Your Balance   126

CHAPTER SEVEN:
Living with Intention: Creating a Home with Soul   142

CHAPTER EIGHT:
Sustainable You: Green Mind, Body, Spirit, and Space   173

CHAPTER NINE:
Holistic Excellence: When It All Comes Together
(or Not) in People, Places, and Things   196

Acknowledgments   216
The Holistic Home Index   217

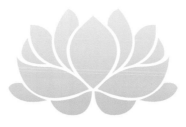

CHAPTER ONE

When Life Hits You on the Head, Listen

"The key to growth is the introduction of higher dimensions of consciousness into our awareness."

—Lao Tzu

Your blood test is abnormal. I'm referring you to a hematologist/oncologist who will do some tests on you. I called him already, and he's expecting to hear from you today." My doctor looked over his bifocals as he handed me a piece of paper with scribbled letters and numbers. This was not what I was expecting from a routine follow-up visit for a bad chest cold. *I am healthy. How can this be? Not me! I'm only thirty-one. I feel great.* I plodded through the next few weeks, alternating between fits of panic and disbelief as I made my way through dozens of tests that included midsection sonograms, radioactive isotopes, and a horrid, botched bone marrow biopsy. Thank God my husband—who was my boyfriend of a year and a half at the time—heard my guttural screams in the waiting room and came bursting through the door to cradle my head while a cylindrical core of my marrow was extracted out of my hip sans anesthesia.

Almost immediately I was given a diagnosis of a rare bone marrow cancer, myelofibrosis, with a recommendation for an "inevitable" bone marrow transplant and a prognosis of four to six years to live. My body felt shell-shocked, and my mind raced with questions from the logical ("What is causing my platelets to over-proliferate?") to the spiritual ("What lesson is this burden trying to teach me?") to the fearful ("How exactly will I be dying?"). I left my job working for a company that represented film directors so I could try to get some answers and get healthier.

A few weeks later, while in a bookstore in downtown Brooklyn, I was rummaging through the health and self-help sections as part of my new life project: Mission Quest for Answers. I bent down to look at some catchy titles with vivid graphics and promises of a hale and hearty life when divine intervention stepped in, in a grand and showy way: a book hit me on my head. Literally hit me on the head. There was no one else even close by that I could have given the evil eye. The book was called *Feng Shui and Health, The Anatomy of a Home: Using Feng Shui to Disarm Illness, Accelerate Recovery, and Create Optimal Health*. I had read many Feng Shui books over the years, but this one seemed quite timely, and *it fell on my head*.

Now, the next part I have often left out when retelling this story. It seems incredibly hokey, but it's true. I looked up to see where it fell from, and the neat, remaining stack was suddenly basked in gold radiance; a ray of sunlight beamed down on the book from a distant window. If this story were reenacted in animation, perhaps at this point a chorus of angels would be singing a joyful and saintly "Ah AHHH" from up above. I had never before received a divine sign in such a literal and blatant way. "Okay. I get it," I told myself. "I should read this book." Just like Oprah said in her final television episode, "Your life is always speaking to you. First in whispers . . . [then] it's like getting a brick upside the head. What are the whispers in your life?" My life was not whispering anymore. It was throwing books at my head. I started listening.

My intuition spoke loudly as I began to see the good and bad connections between my immediate environment and myself. With each recommended change in my home that I made, my space felt more lively, supportive, and purposeful. I started experiencing improvements in several areas of my life. As part of my Mission Quest for Answers, I sought out expert opinions and treatment from the alternative side (kinesiology, aromatherapy, acupuncture, herbs, light therapy) and the mainstream side (three other well-known hematologist/oncologists). Soon it was confirmed that I did not have myelofibrosis, but rather its more gentle and likeable cousin, polycythemia vera! Both are relatively rare and fall under the same umbrella of myelogenous leukemia. And yes, this chronic blood cancer carries its own potential for life-threatening clots and aneurysms, but with a healthy lifestyle and regular medical care—doctor visits, blood tests, and phlebotomies usually every six weeks—a prognosis of a long life can be expected.

Soon after my new diagnosis, I found out the book's author was giving a lecture in New York. I attended and was very impressed with the subject matter and how the author relayed her knowledge. Signing up for her mailing list afterward kept me informed of upcoming classes and training programs, and one day I decided to contact her office to see if I could work for her a couple days a week. She happened to need someone and hired me to help run her office while I went through her training program. Eventually I left to start consulting on my own while studying with other Feng Shui masters, and everything seemed to fall into place. I began to consult, lecture, and teach classes regularly while respectfully being a continuous student myself. I lectured more around the country, wrote about Feng Shui regularly for interior design magazines and blogs, and worked as a Feng Shui and Home & Garden segment host for a popular cable television show. My favorite part, however, was doing consultations for people's homes. My honed and heightened awareness of my surroundings enabled me to be more receptive to the energies that affected my clients.

Through the years, a slow shift occured. I felt a growing need to put the concepts of Feng Shui and energy forth in ways that made sense and in ways that were more personalized for the individual. I looked deeper at all other areas of each client's life. In some regards, I differed greatly from my Feng Shui peers who were steadfastly prescribing crystals, decorative firecrackers, and Foo dogs for their clients or making suggestions like painting their front doors red. What if you don't like the color red? What if you are averse to making your home look like a fast-food Chinese restaurant? I sifted through what works with Feng Shui and what I felt does not. For some, the cultural richness of symbols is quite powerful and might be what they resonate with—and that's fantastic. For others, it's a design nightmare and would just tick them off to have extra tchotchkes around. Red is considered a lucky color in Feng

Shui, but what it comes down to is: if you don't like that color, you are going to hate coming and going through your door every day. And what kind of good energy will that create for you on a daily basis? A simmering undercurrent of negative, that's what. It continued to become clear to me that as miraculous as Feng Shui could be, it needed an update, a staunch edit, and to be integrated as *one part* in the mix of other equally important components. Some concepts I disregard—and I explain why in later chapters—and some I stand by, because I have witnessed profound results for myself and my clients. This book will clarify it all and, most importantly, give a blueprint to uniquely make Feng Shui your own.

CREATING A HOLISTIC HOME

The word *holistic* is a term most people might relate to an alternative health program or an all-inclusive approach to healing. It is defined as balancing and integrating your physical, mental, emotional, and spiritual aspects all together. A Holistic Home is the same concept, but applies to your surroundings and how you can live a healthy, balanced, beautiful life by addressing your mind, body, and spirit in your home and yourself. This approach uses psychology, science, interior design, wellness, green living, and the flow of energy in relatable and at times revolutionary new ways.

This all-inclusive concept was born from my extensive work in Feng Shui but gradually was updated, expanded, and brought into the practical fold of life with a system of addressing the greater whole of who you are. It combines your health, your environment, your relationships, your thinking, and much more as you make the connections between your space and yourself. A Holistic Home connects your mind, body, spirit, and space all together. The mind covers the psychology of how you dwell, subconscious influences, decorating with intention, and how your emotional issues and challenges actually manifest in your space. The physical aspects such as furniture positioning, design elements, green living, wellness, and organization pertain to the body. The spirit covers the invisible energies, the Feng Shui, the atmosphere, your karmic lessons, and the soul of your home. My approach in helping my clients morphed into a much deeper and all-inclusive experience, yet people could easily relate to it. By addressing all the layers from the details to the bigger picture, from the emotions to the décor choices and more, profound transformations occur. Eventually, my consulting grew to large-scale projects, extending to luxury high rises, hotels, hospitals, and retail shops, but the focus is always on how an individual can thrive in each environment from a mind, body, spirit perspective.

A Holistic Home does not have a particular design sensibility like a "Zen look" or an Asian design scheme or a bland beige "organic" look. To an unknowing visitor, it may be a place that inexplicably feels right, where occupants dwell efficiently and the aesthetics all seem to come together. But for you, dear reader, it can also be a home that tremendously elevates your energy, feels solidly balanced, holds meaning, inspires, and supports your health and goals. It begins by setting a goal and focusing your intention, which we will get into shortly. The concept of living a balanced, healthy, and prosperous way of life in accordance with nature has been around for thousands of years as a method of connecting people to heaven and earth.

The more my consultations over the years focused on *all* parts of my clients' lives, the more effective their transformations became. In the beginning, if a consultation concentrated on only paint colors and tips for organization, results would be superficial at best. A consultation that examined, for example, the deeper issues of why you have piles of continuous procrastination appearing as paperwork and laundry and the *real* reasons you are feeling anxious and vulnerable, well, those had life-changing results (as well as no more piles!). By using a dose of logic via psychology and science, combined with an intuitive sense of getting to my clients' core issues, transformations became much more powerful and long-lasting because clients were making changes in ways that aligned with their intellect, psyche, and surroundings. I was inspired to write this book after countless clients of mine relayed their extraordinary stories to me after their consultations. Many of their stories are in this book.

When I am called for a consultation, I know my clients have already taken a big step to welcome change in their lives. The transformation process continues when the connections to their problems are pointed out in their environments. This direct, visual association supports a natural universal flow for an effective change to occur. If you really want to tackle issues in your life that you don't like, I am going to point out, for example, how the fear that is immobilizing you from taking action is physically showing up in your home and then tell you what you can do about it.

Each of these expressions can reveal imbalances, patterns, strengths, weaknesses, or potential problems in specific areas of your life: your chosen neighborhood, the shape of your floor plan, the amount of clutter, loaded symbolism, quality of energy, color choices, furniture positioning, how efficiently you dwell in your home, the balance of the five elements, toxicities in your environment, or electronic device overload. During hundreds of consultations, I clearly saw how these issues show up in many ways. I took notes on each client and their homes. Below are just some of the declarations I have heard from my clients:

- "I just don't feel comfortable in my bedroom and don't like being in there alone."
- "I waste large amounts of time looking for misplaced objects."
- "My children have trouble sleeping and concentrating."
- "I am constantly feeling conflicted."
- "In a room full of people, I often feel alone."
- "I have no energy."
- "The interior design aspects of my home are not coming together, and nothing feels cohesive."
- "I was recently diagnosed with cancer."
- "I want to find a girlfriend, and it's not happening."
- "My husband passed away in the house, and it is hard for me to move on after three years."
- "My career feels stalled and money is scarce."

All these statements are from clients who experienced a transformation once underlying issues were addressed and their recommended adjustments were put in place. As soon as your awareness is heightened, it is easy to see how your immediate environment has an enormous impact on your life. There are definite actions and intentions you can implement in your space that can dramatically influence the opportunities, relationships, finances, and successes you attract.

While on this mission to connect the dots between mind, body, spirit, and design and writing this book, real estate developers, investors, and universities who are on the forefront of future lifestyle trends in design and architecture asked me to be on their teams. Now, with wide-reaching opportunities to work with brilliant creators of new environments, iconic buildings, and future landscapes, I felt it became more important than ever to clarify and edit the misinterpretations, dated notions, and irrelevant concepts of Feng Shui. In addition, the resurgence of Feng Shui that came about in the nineties does not address where we are today. This book will present what works with this ancient art and what does not, as well as delve into future energetic concepts of living. Now, there is definitely an increased consciousness of living that is growing bigger and bigger. From vast organic choices to ever-present "green" options to knowing what farm your meat comes from, people are choosing to live with a more heightened awareness and are ardently making thoughtful selections for a better environment and a better life.

I pledged to put today's version of Feng Shui out there in ways that everyone—no matter where they live, how much money they make, or what their home looks like—could easily understand and implement in order to really *feel* a difference in their spaces and create changes in themselves. But it does take work. Trust that your intimate interiors that you have created—your home—will help guide you in the process as we delve into all areas of your being. You will need to roll up your sleeves and start examining yourself in ways that maybe you never have before. For example, in a consultation, it's common for me to examine both the dark recesses of my clients' minds as well as the symbolic ones in their homes—their closets—to get to the underpinnings of what they fear, what they are hiding, or what they don't want others to see.

MY STORY: BEFORE MY DIAGNOSIS

In the four years leading up to my diagnosis, I was living in a small three-bedroom apartment in Manhattan with my roommate, David. His bedroom was the biggest, mine was a cozy 8 x 10 that could fit only a full-size bed and a small dresser. The third bedroom was even smaller than mine, so we used that as our closet. Knowing what I know now and looking at the floor plan, the potential health issues are quite alarming. An apartment door that upon swinging open would hit the door to the bathroom! (It's called *conflicting doors* in Feng Shui, and it is not lucky to have.) A stove in the kitchen that I could see while lying down on my bed! (Inauspicious, because this configuration can lead to health ailments.) These configurations, I later learned, were not conducive to strengthening my health or stabilizing my blood. This floor plan did not *cause* my health issues, but it certainly did not help support my body in fighting what was brewing.

At the time, I did not know that the entrance to my third-floor walk-up dwelling had such an unfortunate significance in the world of Feng Shui. All I knew was that it was annoying to enter my home if someone left the bathroom door halfway open because both doors would collide, and it would involve an awkward shuffle of arms flailing through small openings on both sides to fully close a door in order to move forward. Later, I discovered the importance of the front door— the energy that flows into your home enters through your front door and then disperses throughout your space. Most times, just entering my door was an exercise in frustration and acrobatics. I later learned to make my front door a prominent feature, making sure it was unencumbered, well lit, and opened freely to welcome all the good chi into my life.

The next home I moved into had a seemingly fine front door. It wasn't hard to open. It was in good condition and even opened into its own respectable entryway. Over the eight years I lived there, I painted it twice, made a mosaic number plate, and installed a peephole. The landlord's bathroom was directly above the front door. After years of a mostly amicable relationship with the landlord, I was surprised when it ended in small-claims court when she refused to return our deposit. My boyfriend and I lovingly tended to every inch of that apartment and always put our own money into upkeep and repairs. I was perplexed how this could happen. Afterward, in the depths of my Feng Shui studies, I learned that a bathroom above the entryway might lead to lawsuits. The judge ruled in our favor and then some, but it left me feeling that the energetic matrix of a house that you are living in can somehow explain the unexplainable. More and more, I realized that while Feng Shui can point out the obvious (a dirty, cluttered home is not a healthy, efficient home), it could also help make sense of the illogical (mysterious illnesses, irrational behavior). Understanding these invisible energies laid the groundwork to comprehend the "spiritual" aspects of living holistically and how to take it even further.

Over the years, I sorted through what clearly works (using the Feng Shui map on your space, tweaking the flow of energy) and took out what does not (feeling obliged to use certain colors or culturally iconic images that you don't connect to; performing particular rituals that might feel forced, toxic, or silly; thinking you have to relocate your front entrance or need to move!). Feng Shui is basically dealing with the energy of a space. When you combine energetic changes with physical and psychological ones, you are tapping into a powerful trifecta of force that can have everlasting effects. Whatever issue you want to work on—optimizing your health, enhancing relationships, finding your calling, or reaching your goals—you will have a surefire way to make it happen by tackling it all, the Holistic Home way. Get ready to delve into your psyche, discover your spiritual lessons, hone your intuition, shed your roadblocks, reach your goals, and create a beautiful and inspiring home along the way.

A TYPICAL CONSULTATION

At least a week before a consultation, I need to receive the client's hand-drawn floor plan and a brief bio or paragraph about any challenges or concerns and where he or she would like to experience a change. When I enter a space, I assess a variety of topics, such as how the energy flows, how efficiently the occupants are dwelling, furniture placement, electrical magnetic fields, the balance of the elements, and the psychology of the chosen décor. As I walk around, I start with the spiritual aspects first—the energetic flow, my intuitive impressions, general atmosphere—and I mentally superimpose the Feng Shui map onto the entire floor plan and also onto each individual room. I ask a lot of questions:

"Tell me, what does this artwork mean to you?"

"Where does each person sit at the dinner table?"

"Who lived here before you?"

Sometimes my questions may seem intrusive. "What is your relationship like with your partner?" Or sometimes they are intuitively based: "Do most of your arguments occur right here?" Each question helps me get to the bottom of the emotional layers that are lying around your home so I can offer specific and effective solutions. Some homes have more emotional garbage lying around than others. I feel it as heaviness or discomfort, depending upon the extent of the emotions that occurred in the space. Other homes can feel somewhat "clean" but might have pockets here and there where arguments, bad dreams, episodes of anxiety, or fear have occurred and are still lingering.

I generally avoid expensive solutions and try to work with what you have. This should not be a costly venture, only an inner tool to improve your life. Often I work with clients throughout the architectural process so that the energetic groundwork, sustainability, and intentions are set from the beginning. No home is holistically "perfect." There are always areas that can be improved and tweaked. It's important that your home be a pure reflection of who you are and not somebody else's personality. In the middle of one consultation, I felt an overwhelming sense that nothing in the house represented the occupant. He said they bought the house fully furnished. The same feeling came over me in another appointment, but that client had a team of persuasive interior decorators whom she allowed to make every design decision for her—from artwork to a group of oddly specific collectibles she had no attachment to. In each consultation, I try to tap into the essence of who the occupants are, and I offer creative solutions to enhance their personal life objectives.

Occasionally there is resistance when certain recommendations are made. This always intrigues me, and I tend to want to get to the bottom of the defiant viewpoint to see where it stems from. Opposition is usually fear-based, and, when properly addressed and dealt with, some of the greatest transformations can take place. An area in your home that may need an energetic adjustment can feel like an open wound. Once pointed out and brought to light, it feels uncomfortable to focus on what is needed to heal. Excuses, resistance, and denial usually occur, and the process may seem exhaustive or insurmountable.

As difficult as this process can sometimes be, it does not stop there. The occupants must work on the recommended adjustments while working on themselves. Just as there is energy in your spatial environment, there is energy flowing in your internal environment—your body. When changes are put into place, the transformed energetic subtleties affect your internal energy or chi. Ways to cultivate your internal chi, such as prayer, visualizations, and meditation, will be discussed in this book.

A consultation can be an emotional process. Nearly every consultation I have done so far—in some way—has been a moving experience. I don't recommend my clients plan any big or important appointments after a consultation because it can be an emotionally exhausting day. I never do more than one per day, because I want to be fresh and ready for each client. I generally avoid doing consultations for family members—it's just too loaded with ingrained dynamics for me to see clearly or effectively convey information they may need to hear in an unbiased way. For a few weeks after every consultation, the client usually has follow-up questions while they make adjustments in their home. Unless there have been major renovations, a move, or a critical life change such as a divorce, illness, death, or birth, I will not return to the home to do another consultation before a year has passed. Some clients don't like this, but this is my rule for a good reason. My goal is to leave my clients (and now you, the readers) with a working understanding of creating a Holistic Home that makes you feel empowered and able to use these tools on your own.

Since I started this journey, I married that wonderful boyfriend. Soon, we will be married thirteen years. We have an incredible almost ten-year-old daughter named

Luchia (notice the chi) and we live in a beautiful home in Brooklyn. My health continues to thrive. I regularly make holistic minded adjustments in my home in accordance with what is needed at the time. Your home should evolve in the same way as you are hopefully evolving. At any given moment, I have at least three home improvement projects I'd like to tackle along with a couple wellness-related aspirations and a few self-improvement goals. As certain goals are met, new adjustments are put in place for future aims, and as new challenges arise or positive changes occur, the environment is aligned to support what may come.

WANTING A CHANGE AND HAVING FAITH IT WILL HAPPEN

I know it may sound simple, but it's important to ask yourself first, "Do I really want to make some changes for the better in my life?" You'd be surprised how many people think they do, but when presented with the step-by-step plan to make it happen, will sabotage it, make excuses, or will not assess themselves honestly. (It's for that reason that I will rarely offer gift certificates for a consultation. *You* have to want it. Not someone else wanting it for you.) Others may simply not believe that a change is possible, and their biggest obstacle is the mistaken belief that it can't happen. For some, change—even for the better—can be scary. It rocks their world, disrupts their routine, and alters their habits. Are you ready to stop making excuses? Are you ready to dig into your inner self and examine your intention and address your fears? Are you ready to open your eyes and see the home that you have created from a different perspective?

Without hesitation, I can honestly say that once you begin to implement this process with openness and intention for the higher good of yourself and others, a change will happen. Once awareness is heightened, connections are realized, chi is cultivated, and physical adjustments are put in place, you'll note energies will shift and transformations will occur. No matter what your issues may be, a mind, body, and spirit approach can be applied to reach goals, become healthier, and feel happier. Sometimes it gets better right away, and other times it gets worse before it gets better.

One thing for sure is that it will not stay the same. "Be prepared for change" is what I usually tell my clients after their consultation ends, because that is when their journey really begins. Now, let's begin yours.

CHAPTER TWO

Starting Clean: De-cluttering Your Mind, Body, and Spirit

"Knowing is not enough; we must apply. Willing is not enough; we must do."

—Johann von Goethe

An acupuncturist reads pulses. A doctor reads X-rays. And I read your home—because in every case, that's where I find the clearest facts about your life—in heaps of unfolded laundry, in unsorted mail, in piles deep within your closet. In particular, your clutter reveals more about you than you might realize—and not just that you don't have the right Container Store products either, but your deepest fears, anxieties, and roadblocks. Before you and I get into the thrill of activating some tremendous changes in your space and yourself, you must first clear away all your garbage. That means addressing every bit of negative clutter, from the dusty piles of unread magazines by your bed to the self-doubt running through your head. First, we are going to tackle the area where negative clutter shows up the most, and it is the command control center for your life—it's the gray matter between your ears.

A de-cluttered mind is free of all the various forms of mental, emotional, and spiritual clutter preventing you from open, clear thinking. Clutter in all its forms is negative, stuck, unhealthy energy. Holistically clearing your mind allows you to shed the baggage, embrace the good, live in the present, and have faith that the "bad" will eventually reveal itself as a vital life lesson for the better. Once that occurs, you can easily hone your intention, clarify your goals, and learn to use reflection with cerebral action to move from a negative space to a positive outcome.

In every chapter of this book, ways to achieve the changes you desire will be offered by using the mind, body, and spirit all together. Because, for example, if you were to just deal with the action and physical aspects (body) of clutter and throw out all your junk or install some file cabinets, or hire a professional organizer to do all your work, sure, your home might look better temporarily, but the real reasons why you have physically accumulated stuff (mind) and the unseen energies (spirit) connected to it all would not help support the change. Your home would be back to how it looked—or worse—in no time. Once you get into the habit of addressing all three of these parts of who you are, you will naturally look for ways to adjust and unite your mind, body, and spirit in relation to your environment when you desire other changes as well.

First, I will delve into the tools you will need, ways to shed mental clutter and how to identify the deeper meaning of your physical and spiritual clutter, and will offer tips to keep it all in check. Once the interiors of your mind and your home are free of clutter, you are more open to unleash your energy and sharpen your personal focus, and are ready to begin the *whole* transformation that you will be experiencing with this book.

THE MIND AND CLUTTER

Mind clutter is negative thoughts, scattered thinking, self-doubts, cynicism, indecisiveness, procrastination, worry, and fear-based thinking. You can de-clutter your mind by having a clear focus of your daily goals, specific intentions, and a sense of inner strength. Think of all the clarity that you'll have with your decision-making and how your creativity, intuition, or focus will thrive without the mental chaos that is an inevitable part of your busy life. Meditation, mantras, mental exercises, prayer, and a positive, new shift in perspective are your tools to make it happen.

MEDITATION

Meditation is a great way to ground and focus oneself, reduce stress, and develop calmness. When chaos erupts around you, if your inner core is uncluttered and unwavering, you will have a boost over others who may crumble under pressure or slip into unhealthy behaviors. You will have a grounded sense of certainty to "keep calm and carry on." Daily meditations can help you maintain a clear focus that enables you to keep the mental clutter at bay. Meditation can lower blood pressure, increase deeper levels of relaxation, and greatly increase your levels of concentration. If meditation is new to you, start with just giving yourself five minutes per day to sit quietly, focus on your breath, and do nothing. Gradually build up to more time where stillness is the goal and a mind void of chatter is the outcome.

A PERSONAL MANTRA

The Sanskrit translation for *mantra* means "instrument of thought," and it is believed to create transformation within. Mantras help focus your mind when it is scattered and help dispel negative thoughts. Try starting the day with a personal mantra that you say to yourself nine times as you prepare for your day. Sit down with paper and pen and try to come up with your own personal mantra. Below are some examples you can modify to come up with one that feels best to you. Say it in your head, say it quietly, or sing it loud and proud.

Today I am calm, assured, confident, and flowing with certainty.
I am taking into my life only what is absolutely needed.
I am productive, resourceful, and wise in all tasks, choices, and statements I make.
Today I will focus on seeing the positive, feeling the gratitude, and being at peace.

PRAYER

Whether you are in a church, lying in bed, holding others' hands or your own, prayer is a personal way to increase your chi, set your goals, and instill gratitude within yourself. The important thing is that your prayer comes from the heart and that you hold faith that your desires are being heard. When most people pray, they are either praying for themselves, others, or sharing praise and thanks. Whatever God, deity, angel, or universal force you resonate with, try including a prayer for yourself, asking for peace of mind, clarity, compassion, and strength to overcome whatever obstacles are put your way. Pray for all the negative clutter in your life to be revealed, released, and eliminated. Pray for the insight to see the truth behind the reasons holding you back and the strength to create the ideal life you desire.

GO NEGATIVE TO GET TO THE POSITIVE

A holistic mind means attracting the positive. Believe it or not, you can get there by visiting your dark side. By acknowledging the issue you want to change while *holding the intention for constructive growth*, you are in a state of progress, which is positive energy. Stagnant, stuck energy is the clutter of your soul. Forward movement, whether it is the act of cleaning out a junk drawer or saying a mantra for personal development, is all positive energy. Positive energy owns up to the negative and uses it as a tool to move forward. Positive energy begets itself. If you are emanating positivity, it will shine back on you. People who radiate negativity will be repelled from you.

Another way to utilize your dark side for all it's worth is to visit it quickly now and then to either realize how far you have come or how lucky you are. Use it as a reality check, and it will also increase compassion or gratitude in your life. When you are in the midst of hardship, try to visit an *even darker place* of a scenario that could be much worse. This concept may feel counterintuitive at first, but it can be a strong power-shifter while in a bad place. Sit with that feeling for a few minutes. Then, feel the gratitude in knowing that is not your situation. Allow your focus to be on visualizing a shining, healthy, ideal outcome. Remain steady with your vision, and remember not to get stuck in the dark—you are only dropping in for a quick visit to get your bearings and move on. Don't let the mental clutter—the doubting, sabotaging, cynical chatter—get in the way. These fear-based doppelgangers are not your friends and need to be tossed out just like yesterday's newspapers and those pants that have not fit you for ages. By going darker momentarily, the light is brighter when you let it in. Let it shine.

Most people have difficulty seeing the sunshine in the midst of a seemingly pitch-black hole. One way to cope with this is by finding comfort in complaining briefly about things that don't go your way. Yep, that's right. Complaining. But you must follow the specific formulas below of *How to De-Clutter Your Mind* and *Be Clear in What You Want* so you don't become an irritable Debbie Downer or a toxic energy vampire but, instead, a Holistically Balanced You. Here's how:

HOW TO DE-CLUTTER YOUR MIND

When the world seems against you or you have become your own worst enemy, go ahead and talk about it. Speak up and say it out loud. But instead of just bitching and moaning, get to the root cause of your complaint. Be specific with what is really bothering you. Let it all out. (Choose the receiver of your diatribe carefully. Usually a trusted best friend or empathetic family member is best.) Look at it as purging the clutter in your mind to make room for the positive. Holding on to negative mental clutter is not healthy, and having only a "send light and love" approach is not practical or effective on its own. There are many self-help books out there now that talk about reveling in the love and sending love and light as the panacea for all. Light and love are vital in the equation, and will come later as the beautiful icing on the cake in this process, but without addressing the fundamental aspect of your clutter and taking action to eliminate it in a realistic and truthful way, it will always remain. No matter how much love and light you throw at it, it will endlessly endure. You must take action—both mentally and physically—before you can light it up and smother it with good intentions and release it. First, you need to identify your own personal mental clutter.

Identifying the Source

We already identified some common mental clutter as negative thoughts, scattered thinking, self-doubts, cynicism, indecisiveness, procrastination, worry, and fear-based thinking. So, what is yours? When you go through these, is there one that resonates with you? Recognize what is polluting your mind at the moment. When you go to a dark place, what is leading you there? What occupies the majority of your negative thoughts? Write it down or say it out loud. This simple act of specifically identifying your type of mental clutter and saying it out loud can be powerful because you are calling it out. You are not allowing it to have a secret power over you. By acknowledging it—you can also write about it in a journal or shout it from your rooftop—you are beginning to release it. Once you acknowledge it, as tempting as it may feel, don't dwell on it or revisit it. Practice using your tools of meditation, mantras, or prayer while *simultaneously* tackling all the physical clutter in your space. If the same negative mental clutter attempts to seep in down the road, don't give it the precious real estate of your thoughts. Acknowledge, visualize, act, and release. Remember to move forward by focusing on a positive visualization of your specific outcome.

Be Clear in What You Want

You must imagine your ideal outcome in precise detail. Often clients will tell me things like, "Well, I want abundance in my life!" Abundance can show up on your hips. Abundance can manifest in your bills. Abundance can mean even more clutter in your surroundings. When you are focused on a clear and definite outcome, you are helping the Universe deliver it to you without the clutter. When you hold that specific visualization as you implement your mind, body, and spirit tips while you are making adjustments in your environment, your outcome will be much more powerful and effective. Know that *you* hold the power to create the transformation you desire. It's okay if you can't picture how it will happen, just have faith that it *will*. Expect the results you want. Know, with certainty, without wavering, that your desired outcome will happen. In addition to holding this mental picture while going through each chapter and making your holistic adjustments, try to start carrying these thoughts with you continuously throughout your day. Your own affirmative thoughts will begin to attract similar situations, interactions, or experiences that are in alignment with your goals. This is not wishful thinking. This is actively choosing to harness your universal birthright of attaining beneficial energy and ideal opportunities in your life. Right now you are holding a book in your hands that is a direct result of unwavering intention and an inexplicable knowing from deep within my soul that this book would get published. There was never a doubt in my mind—even though many others certainly doubted it.

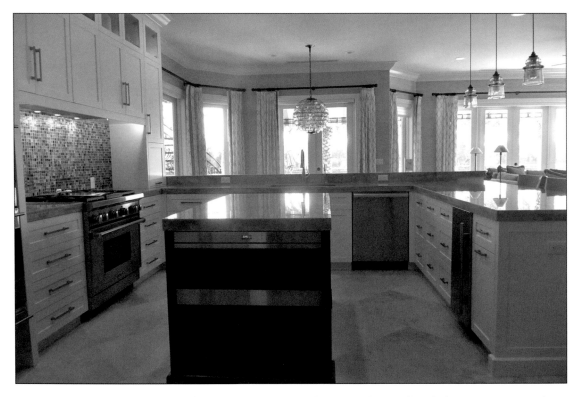

When you're in need of clarity, a great exercise to do is to clear off and clean your immediate surfaces. The act itself helps you focus, and the clear planes psychologically enhance your concentration.

Holistic Body Tip

As you go through your cleaning-out process, vividly visualize your desired end result. Imagine how your home looks: neat and tidy, with everything around you in sharp, crisp, clear focus. Every item has a place. Imagine how your home smells: fresh like a spring day, as if you just finished a deep cleaning or filled the space with your favorite fragrant flowers. Imagine how your home feels: the atmosphere feels lighter. You are only surrounded by the stuff you absolutely love that makes your heart say "Yes!" and fills you with vitality.

MY STORY: MY FATHER, GENE BENKO

Four years ago, my father was in the hospital in intensive care after two emergency colorectal surgeries in a row went awry. He was getting worse quickly and had to endure yet another surgery to save his life. At the end of this harrowing day, Mom and I went back to the B&B we were staying at near the hospital. We hadn't eaten all day and were exhausted. It was Christmas Day. No restaurants in the area were open—not even the hospital cafeteria. We shared one thin chocolate wafer that was left on our pillow and called the ICU every hour throughout the night to get updates on his condition. We cheered and hugged when one nurse reported that his temperature came down one degree.

My father is the most positive being I have ever known. Even though he suffered greatly and felt fear and defeat during this ordeal, he simply kept persevering and beat all odds to survive. He never gave up and even managed to cheer up others along the way. Negative energy sucks you in, spirals you down, and makes you unhealthy. Positive energy nods to the terrible, yet moves through it to gain strength and a fresh perspective. When negative clutter entered his mind, he acknowledged it and then powered through, allowing his current set of goals to be the focus. My father had to go to a rehab facility after weeks in the hospital to regain strength just to walk. During this time, he told me, "If they want me to do five ball tosses, I'll do ten!" He set goals and surpassed them. My family did everything we could to help speed his recovery. (In this case, it was procuring a signed Judge Judy photograph and even getting Judge Judy to leave him a personal voice mail message of encouragement, which he listened to over and over.) Months later, my father, in his seventies, got back to leading a productive, generous, and thoughtful life. He continued to get dressed up in his suits and go to the office—the very first place I ever Feng Shui'd. (My dad was my first willing "client" eons ago when I was in my Feng Shui training.)

Sometimes I do quick drive-bys in my mind by revisiting dark moments like that Christmas Day. I see myself in the surgical waiting room, fraught with fear and desperation. Then, I quickly go to where I am now and let the focus be on how far my dad has come. I marvel in the progress he has made and relish in the current, positive state of his health. This is a surefire way to spontaneously generate an abundance of gratitude or a rush of optimism within yourself. Think back to a dark time in your life. Or even a time when things were not going as you hoped. Chances are, with time and space for reflection, a positive outcome can be found, a lesson can be learned, or an "everything happens for a reason" might be felt. The more growth you have experienced since that moment, the more the dark spot acts like your teacher.

Exactly two years later, while I was writing my dad's story in the paragraph above, my mom calls me and tells me that Dad has had a setback and is going to the hospital for tests and possible surgery. He's a highly complex case, so he gets rushed to the same specialized hospital far away from home. Again it's Christmas morning, and I leave my husband and daughter, with presents under the tree, to rush to Dad's side in the hospital. Dad never looked better. His hair was perfectly combed, he was sitting up in a chair, smiling and talking with his trademark strong and booming voice. In a private moment later with my mom, walking to the elevator, she tells me, "His spirit is so much bigger than the body that holds him together." The doctors were doing all they could to avoid surgery, so a battery of tests explored other options. Meanwhile, doctors and nurses from all over the hospital who remember him from two years ago came to visit him and tell him what an inspiration he is. Some had thought about him often since his last ordeal in the hospital; others had read published medical stories about his miraculous recovery.

My dad attributes his tenacious optimism simply to a love of life. "It's not that I don't go to these dark places. I do. I just focus on other things." He tells me often that he feels like a lucky man. I've read enough studies to know that if you *think* you are lucky, you are more likely to experience luck. Perhaps my father's greatest tip to share is that he lives his life feeling thankful for each day, rather than feeling disappointed for what is not in it.

When my father was back in the hospital on Christmas, he allowed himself to feel disappointment for the crappy situation he was in; he briefly imagined an unfavorable outcome, acknowledged some pain he was feeling, but then he released it. A cloud of pain, fear, and angst went out the window and was released into the clouds above. The frequent, hovering medical helicopter blades on the roof above him chopped it all up. Then his main focus became planning the details for a family cruise to Alaska and walking out of the hospital in great shape. Both happened. He left the hospital with pep in his step. A year and seven months later, Dad was feeling on top of the world—literally and metaphorically—while standing on top of the Mendenhall Glacier in Juneau, Alaska, with the entire family around him, loving life.

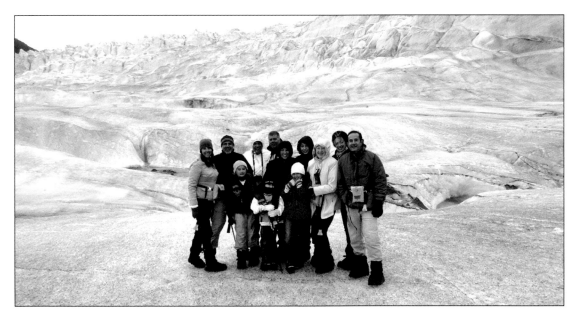

Mendenhall Glacier, Alaska. Mom and Dad are in the white hoods, surrounded by immediate family.

A holistic mind means being crystal clear with your thoughts and goals and knowing how to harness the dark to catapult you into the light. This Yin and Yang cerebral balance of the wits enables the most positive growth to happen. If you follow this formula, you will be more productive, more positive, happier, lighter, and more at peace. You will be capable of getting rid of the physical junk around you because you are clear and focused and will realize the connections between the stacks of old newspapers and the lack of zest you feel about sticking to your New Year's resolutions. You might even start to feel lucky.

LIVING IN THE NOW

Clutter creates stagnant energy. When you are stagnant, there is little growth happening, and you will tend to either live in the past and feel sad or live in the future and feel anxious. By clearing the clutter—internally and externally—you are allowing yourself to live holistically in the *now*. When you have mental clutter, you are preoccupied with negative chatter, lists, doubt, distractions, and worries that are prohibiting you from being in the moment. When you have physical clutter, you can easily feel overwhelmed, exhausted, defeated, unproductive, and out of control. When you have spiritual clutter, you can subconsciously feel weighted down, irrational, emotional, and unstable. All of these negative feelings imprison you in a clutter rut, which keeps you stuck in either the past or future. You cannot fully live and enjoy life in the moment when you have mental, physical, and spiritual clutter within you and around you.

KAREN: MENDING FURNITURE AND HER SUBCONSCIOUS

Karen contacted me for a consultation because she felt overwhelmed, out of control emotionally, and desperate for help. Her bio indicated that she was disorganized with telling information such as "I often can't focus . . . it takes me a long time to get moving on things" and "I rarely have people over." She revealed she was "often down in the dumps" and felt run-down. A chaotic environment can easily lead to frustration, a lack of concentration, and instability. Procrastinating and feeling overwhelmed are significant side effects of disorganization. It is definitely harder to get ready, get motivated, or get inspired in an unsystematic, disorderly home. If Karen was having difficulty focusing and her physical space was in disarray, her mind space would be, too.

I knocked on her door, and after several minutes, the door opened, but I could not see Karen. Karen was behind the door, waiting for me to enter. She semi-hid herself there so I could squeeze my way in. Piles of junk, trash, newspapers, clothes, and broken pieces of furniture formed waist-high mountains, which were bisected by narrow paths that formed walkways from specific areas: kitchen to bathroom to couch. And couch to bathroom to bed. The air smelled stale and felt thick and heavy as if stepping over her threshold projected me into a different humidity zone. The simple act of breathing in that cramped space felt more labored than the unthinking process it regularly is. Clutter causes energy to stagnate. Instead of circulating in a healthy, clean flow, the energy accumulates in a weighted-down form, which, inexorably, leads to low energy, lethargy, and a sense of feeling overwhelmed.

Karen could only clear off a small space on the couch where we both had to sit super close. We talked for the next two hours. I knew that disorganization to such an extreme level stemmed from mental clutter challenges and hoped that Karen would be open to the process of allowing herself to get to some core issues in our short time together. I knew it would be tough. Clutter, in all its forms, is intensely intertwined with the psyche. Dismantling this tormented way of living does not start by removing the physical stuff: it begins by getting to the root of the psychological problem. If you collect in an unhealthy, excessive manner (and an overloaded medicine cabinet can qualify you for that) you *can* become clutter-free forever. You can also live in a space that enables you to have clarity, focus, drive, inner peace, and a new, efficient way of existing. If you try to begin this process without holistically addressing your mind first and just start tossing, not only will it not work, but clutter will also return, twice as much as before. The cerebral issues must be addressed so you can you realize the true reasons behind your accumulating nature and make an effective change. Only when you honestly identify these reasons and work on them can the letting-go begin. Eventually, when you start to get rid of both the mental and physical junk, you will find that the more you do it, the easier it is to let go, and a new, freer emotion will result.

After an emotional session of releasing her story, Karen walked me through the apartment, and at a snail's pace, we discussed the meanings behind her possessions. Stacks of newspapers and magazines created towers of dormant energy. This can contribute to laziness and hopelessness. When you have piles of clutter like this, you are creating energetic anchors of malaise, which prohibit new opportunities and experiences from entering your life. When asked why she did not throw out used magazines, Karen did not have an answer. Some people need old magazines for reference, such as recipes or interior design inspirations. If that's you, I recommend tearing out only the articles that pertain to your specific needs, sliding them into clear plastic sleeves, and storing them in a binder. You can shrink a year's subscription into one medium-sized binder, keeping only what you absolutely need.

Karen had a habit of collecting broken furniture with the hope that she would one day find the time to get it repaired. She would pick up furniture from garbage piles at the curb or from her apartment building's basement where there was an ongoing heap, discarded from the occupants of the building. A couple of the residents in the building who were friendly with her and aware of Karen's problem had begun to put signs on their items: "FREE CHAIR—EXCEPT FOR YOU, KAREN!" Items that are broken, in need of repair, or not functioning properly are considered clutter. When I inquired about what was going on for her emotionally when she brought home the busted chair, the broken mirror, and the dresser with no drawers, she went silent. After a while, she said she was dealing with her mother's illness each time—either coming or going from visiting her or feeling overly occupied with thoughts of her condition. As her mother was diagnosed with a terminal illness and getting progressively worse, Karen would bring home more and more broken furniture. Then, I saw the recognition in her eyes as she began to see the connections I pointed out between her life issues and her environmental ones. With each piece of furniture she brought home, she carried the hope that she could fix it, make it better, and bring it back to its glory days with the same hope that she held for her mother. Instead, Karen's broken, untouched, and unused items strewn in her surroundings were subconscious reminders of failure and unfulfilled dreams. The excess stuff insulated her from the harsh outside world that took her mother's health.

When immersed in an emotionally charged situation where you feel you have no control, it's common to want to exert control over other areas. Realizing this connection was a powerful moment for Karen. A major and abrupt turning point occurred because she was both aware and willing to make a change at that moment. Maybe you, too, have had a moment in your life like this. Like when you suddenly realized the not-good-for-you-relationship you were in was wrong—even though people had been telling you for ages—but something finally clicked internally and you never looked back. In dealing with your clutter, if you are ready to make a change and able to make the real emotional connections between your accumulations to the barriers that hold you back, a transformation is sure to follow.

DEALING WITH NOSTALGIA

When you surround yourself with items from your past, it's easy to live in the past. I've been in homes where not even a single placemat was changed over the last thirty years. And the occupants' views on life seemed just as dusty and antiquated as their thirty-year-old placemats. Are you keeping items because they were bequeathed to you, and you feel a sense of obligation? Are you holding on to that ugly frame that you secretly hate but can't bear to throw out because it was a gift? Give it away to someone you think might enjoy it. Give it to charity. Get it out of your home. One friend of mine donates her unwanted gifts to Chinese auctions and has great satisfaction knowing that someone will get an item they actually want.

It's okay to have some mementos, as long as you carefully and honestly examine the origin of association attached to it. One way to begin to get some control with over-acquiring is when you first see an object, to be aware of what goes through your mind. See each item as one of two things: either it lifts your energy or it depletes it.

"Well, what about neutral items like perfectly fine pots and pans?" Karen asked.

"Their purpose is to help nourish you, so that is uplifting. But don't let an excessive quantity be depleting," was my reply. Once you determine what is left that is uplifting, then evaluate the quantity.

In addressing Karen's sense of feeling overwhelmed, highly emotional, and stuck in the past, I asked her to point out the items in her home that represented hope, peace of mind, or inspiration. She quickly answered that her rescue dogs gave her all those feelings. Earlier in the consultation, she had said that she would have a hard time getting rid of things because it reminded her of certain events in her life or significant people that she never wanted to forget. But when Karen began to tell the nostalgic stories, none of them was necessarily heartwarming: "This sewing machine was from a grandmother who never really liked me. She was always crabby and mean and when she died, my mother gave it to me." Upon closer reflection, she realized that she never really did like it after all, but it represented a sense of familiarity that merged into a sense of obligation to keep. I recommended Karen hang up pictures of her dogs instead.

Holistic Mind Tip:

One of the most common occurrences for accumulating clutter is keeping items out of a sense of obligation or just because they are familiar. You should *never* feel obligated to choose to surround yourself with objects you don't even like. The energetic manifestations of that subconscious feeling will snowball every time, and you'll never know why you're walking around so angry and bitter. If you don't honestly love it, let it go.

Next up: "This dresser was the only thing I had after an ex moved out on me," Karen said.

"You are holding on to energy that does not serve you well," I told her. Her bio detailed the extent of the bad relationship, and I felt it was important for her to try to take an objective look at the connection. "This item does not honor who you are. It only serves as a reminder of a bad relationship and depletes your confidence. Get rid of it," I told her.

In the depths of a dark and distant pile from the corner, I pulled out several bits and pieces and asked Karen to tell me why she had them. Every object I pulled out, Karen had an emotional response and claimed the item as "very meaningful." If an object is very meaningful to you, it should be properly showcased and displayed in a way that honors its significance. The butterfly that she caught with her father before he died could be mounted and framed and hung on the wall or placed in a treasure box and stored in a drawer. Karen was using her chaotic surroundings to distract herself from real issues she felt she did not have the courage to tackle. Now that she was aware of how it energetically held her, she said she wanted to be set free. Due to the enormity of Karen's issues and how they had physically manifested over the years, she needed to take small steps to minimize the potential shock, which might lead to a rebound of clutter coddling.

If you genuinely desire a change in your life, once the connections are made, you will continue submerging yourself in a sea of disorganization unless the following five steps occur.

The Key to Transformation:

- You truly want to make a change.
- Identify the core issues.
- Take physical and mental action to eliminate the clutter.
- Associate a strong visualization of the unwanted emotion onto the objects you are removing.
- Continually work with this new way of being so that it becomes your natural lifestyle.

IDENTIFYING WHY YOU ACCUMULATE

Keep in mind that it does take *work* to examine the root of your accumulation issues. For many, this lifestyle offers a sense of solace and protection. It can feel insulating from the harsh world outside, which may not have been good to some people. There are many other reasons why people hoard items or even simply just accumulate mounds of clutter in particular areas. Mostly, the reasons stem from varying forms of fear. Fear of not having enough causes people to accumulate.

Perhaps you grew up in a depression or grew up very poor, and now you may be trying to protect yourself from ever feeling without again. Fear of forgetting the past or who you are or fear of being vulnerable all lead to a pack-rat mentality. Fear of failure or even fear of success is a common reason for clutter.

When it comes time to release, more fear comes up. Accumulators are usually scared of getting rid of their objects because of the fear of losing a part of themselves; losing a memory, losing money, losing their identity, losing their creativity, or losing security. We will discuss how fear shows up and how to tackle it in chapter 7.

If you are looking around your home now and realize that you have some clutter issues, hopefully the table on the following pages will help you get in touch with the real reasons why. Not, "I'm just too busy to deal with the paperwork." We are all busy. That is the biggest and lamest excuse there is. You can do better than that. I'm looking for something like this: "My drive for perfection is preventing me from sorting through these piles in the precise and thorough way I feel is necessary." Bingo.

Once you have identified your type of clutter, ask yourself the core questions to help make the physical changes. With this new insight, shift the picture in your mind's eye as you take the action necessary to banish the buildup in your surroundings. Start slow at first, focusing more on the emotional aspects as you sift through a small stack every day for a week. When you drop the unwanted paperwork into the shredder and carry it out on recycling day, visualize that you are really carrying out a big bag of self-imposed restrictions to the curb. Whatever your underlying root issue is—fear, worry, denial—visually attach that to the unwanted objects you are letting go. Add a verbal confirmation as you do this, such as, "I am releasing my unhealthy need for control.

I am freeing myself of critical judgment, which no longer serves me." Continue this exercise on a daily basis every time you throw out the garbage or give items away.

Types of Fear/Clutter		
Type of Fear	**How it Shows Up**	**Solution**
Fear of Success/ Low Self-Esteem	Artwork or mirrors that are unintentionally hung too high, leaving you subconsciously feeling like you can never measure up, are indications of low self-esteem and a fear of success.	As a rule of thumb, artwork and mirrors should be 60 inches from center to floor. Remind yourself you are setting realistic expectations for yourself, while you bring everything to eye level. It's a fresh start for your self-esteem.
Fear of Failure	Piles of procrastination and avoidance show up in the form of paperwork, clothes, odds and ends, or unfinished to-do lists.	You can tackle this by focusing on being confident with your decisions as you tackle the hardest tasks first on your to-do list. Being organized and clutter-free will help you focus on your strengths and accomplishments.
Fear of Uncertainty	When you have a desire to insulate yourself with an excessive amount of belongings, leading to stockpiling and hoarding, you are battling a fear of the unknown.	Remind yourself you can't find true security in items you can buy. Hoarding communicates to your subconscious that you are in need, a message that can become a self-fulfilling prophecy.
Fear of Commitment	Putting off hanging artwork, selecting paint colors, updating décor, unpacking boxes, and procrastinating on any big-ticket purchases are indications that you are hesitant to commit.	You can start to combat your fear of commitment by making a list of only the things you don't want in your home (the color red, southwest décor, clutter, etc.). This creates boundaries while opening possibilities to follow your instincts. Create a budget you can afford, and make your choices when you are in a good mood—not stressed or under pressure.

Types of Fear/Clutter *(Continued)*		
Type of Fear	**How it Shows Up**	**Solution**
Fear of Change	When your décor hasn't been updated since you moved in and you haven't freshened up a single item in eons, you are suffering from a fear of change.	To begin the process of transforming, start by moving your bed or desk. A new perspective from these two main pieces of furniture can help you literally and figuratively see things differently. Make sure you don't have your back to the door. You want to feel empowered and be able to see who is entering, not vulnerable or easily startled.
Fear of Losing Control	A meticulously ordered home where anxiety lurks with even the slightest possibility of chaos, disorder, or violated house rules indicates a fear of losing control.	A looser, forgiving home is a more relaxed and joyful place to be. When messes occur, repeat to yourself, "Go with the flow," for five long exhales.

THE BODY AND CLUTTER

We covered mental clutter and how to identify and deal with it; now let's move on to body clutter, which is physical clutter. It's all the actual stuff stagnating your space because it serves no purpose. There is only value in the things you use regularly. Clutter is stuck, unhealthy, unproductive, draining energy. It makes you feel tired and exhausted. It can also show up as an accumulation of extra pounds. It makes you late for appointments and unable to find items when you really need them. Piles of paperwork and clothes, outgrown toys, knickknacks, dusty collectibles, junk, broken and unused items—even dirt and grime are clutter.

Discover what your go-to excuses are. Ask yourself the deeper questions related to your excuse. Now is not the time to try to justify, blame, or give more excuses.

Be honest. No one is judging you. As you take the necessary action, go at your own pace. Start with a junk drawer or a medicine cabinet and then work your way up to a closet. After that, continue on room by room. You will find, however, that the more you let go, the easier it is to do. Assess what is working for you and what is not. Set goals. Ask yourself, "What items are most essential to me?" Purge. Throw out anything broken, unused, or forgotten. If you have not used the item in over a year, toss it. Give your stuff away. Give to charity and get a tax deduction. If you think a friend might have a need for it, give it to them. Have a yard sale. You might be surprised how much money you can make in a couple hours of selling unwanted items.

HOW TO PHYSICALLY DE-CLUTTER

For Karen, I suggested she start letting go in small steps by releasing the pieces that were in need of the most mending that she didn't have the strongest emotional attachment to. She wrote down a step-by-step plan of furniture removal goals that I suggested over the course of the next month. If your entire home is jam-packed with clutter, start by having one room designated as clutter-free. Let this space be your clean and organized refuge where absolutely no clutter is allowed in. When feeling mentally cluttered, go in there and tune in to the differences that you feel while in this clear space. Let this room be your inspiration to continue the process. Do not bring anything else into your home for at least one week. Go through each room systematically, asking yourself the questions on the following page, and then attach the underlying emotion to what you are tossing.

Questions to Ask Yourself

If you are not sure what your home reflects, start with a single room, go through each object, and honestly ask yourself the following questions:

- Does this style really reflect me?
- Does this represent who I am right now and who I want to be?
- Does this item lift my spirits?
- Do I use it regularly?
- Does it make me feel good when I see it/use it or do I feel bitter or full of regret?
- Do I absolutely love this room?

Attach an Emotion

As you clean out your space, it's important to attach the underlying root emotion to the stuff you're tossing. For example, suppose you have determined that you accumulate because of the death of your parent at an early age. Your clutter represents a layer of protection and safety. While you're removing the clutter, visualize that you're throwing out the emotion of feeling scared and unprotected. There it lies in a black garbage bag at the curb now. Say good-bye.

As you continue the cleaning-out process, try saying your personal mantra as you go along or come up with a new one. "My belongings do not define me. I am safe. I am strong. I am clear in all my decisions. I am surrounding myself with only the things I use and love."

When the time feels right, move on to other emotions you would like to get rid of and attach them to everything you throw out. Even in small ways—as you clean out the refrigerator or empty wastebaskets—attach your undesirable traits of mental clutter to them as you toss. For me, I just left a big, black bag of worry by the curb, and I feel better already. By attaching an unwanted emotion to clutter while holding a positive visualization for the outcome you desire, transformations will be easier. In addition to removing what is no longer needed, focus on what is important to you.

Now you know what you don't want. So let's focus on what you do want. This systematic blend of mind, body, and spirit supports a more effective and complete transformation.

As you go through this process, try to eliminate whatever does not serve you well; that means anything that lowers your mood, that you haven't used in one year, or that you genuinely don't love. Maybe you grew out of it or you said you would fix it someday, but now it's years later. If you are keeping furniture from a departed loved one just because it was bequeathed to you, but you don't really like it, give it away! Every time you look at that object, you are bound to feel some underlying resentment. Imagine that emotion building up every day and manifesting into other unhealthy emotions. It's time to let go and give yourself a fresh slate. When you do this assignment, keep the intention that you are creating a space that will move, inspire, comfort, heal, or relax you.

Holistic Body Tip

Don't multitask. By concentrating on one mission at a time, you're making the most efficient use of time. It is easy to kid oneself and believe otherwise, but most mistakes, delays, and confusions happen when we sacrifice our concentration by spreading our attention in numerous directions. Multitasking leads to scattered energy, and eventually projects take longer to accomplish. Generally, try to keep a steady stream of focus on one de-cluttering task until it is complete and then move to another.

After the completion of each organizational task, be mindful of how you feel. Sit with the feeling of accomplishment and relish feeling productive. Let this new focus be the momentum to bring you to another bigger project.

LIVING WITH A SLOB

If you are organized, but other people you live with are not, try to integrate a system that works for their individual sense of style and needs. Make baskets or contemporary leather boxes available as decorative ways to hold things. Loose papers, coins, keys, and often-used items are best placed in covered containers that are easy to access. Label the underside of the lid as to what should go in there. Encourage your partner to stick to the new storage system by surprising them with treats or notes of encouragement in their containers when they start to get the hang of it. If at first they don't put the item in its new home, do it for them. Soon enough they'll ask, "Have you seen my wallet?" Tell them for the third time, "It's in the brown leather box on your dresser where it belongs." Out of habit, they'll eventually start to put it there themselves. Be dependable with your own organizational system so that your organizationally challenged partner will hopefully learn through osmosis or by consistency. After your home is organized, ask them how they feel in a clean space versus an unmanageable one. Hopefully they will read this book and begin to align themselves on the side of order with you.

LIVING WITH A NEAT FREAK

The clutter bug and the neat freak actually have a couple things in common. First, each is coming from a place of fear or imbalanced conditioning, and second, task completion can be delayed for both. We already established the fear issues that cause people to be highly unorganized or excessive collectors, so the top fears for the neat freaks are not being in control, fear of change, or fear of mistakes. When you attempt to control every aspect of an environment, you lose the essence of living in the present and acting spontaneously. Also, such high standards tremendously stress out everyone in the household. As usual, the key to living harmoniously is balance. It is not a sin to let the dishes pile up if it means you get to spend extra time with your children or take a walk with your partner. Being orderly and organized is about creating a home that allows you to be the best you can be. Your home should be a place that allows you to relax in the way that you desire. Everyone is different, and all will have diverse levels of acceptance with organization. Try to operate on what makes you intuitively feel good about yourself and the expectations you hold for others.

Holistic Body Tip

Drink lots of water as you purge your home of your clutter. It's your body's cleansing tool. Water helps remove toxins from the body and makes you feel fresh—like your home will feel.

DEALING WITH KIDS' CLUTTER

When a photographer came to my home to take some pictures of me, she kept looking around in disbelief, saying, "But where is all your crap?" I asked her, like what? "Newspapers, magazines?" My reply, "E-subscriptions help keep that at bay. For other hands-on reading material, I have a rule: newspapers go to the recycling bin at the end of the day, magazines can stay only for a few weeks." I also tried to explain that I don't allow "crap" into my life. I simply will not put up with it—whether that "crap" is toxic relationships, negative behavior, or not addressing issues directly when they need to be. If you have low-energy–value crap around you (e.g., day-old newspapers), you are dwelling in a place convoluted with an additional layer of nonsense. Try to evaluate the energetic value of the items that surround you because that directly affects the situations and relationships you bring in to your life. Low-energy items magnetize a low-energy life. The end goal is to keep the crap away and the sacred close.

When we got to the subject of managing our kids' clutter, the photographer said, "But I will never throw out *any* of my son's artwork because that would mean I'm a bad mom." *Hmm.* If you don't realize that it's your love and guidance that define you as a mom, then it will be hard to convince you otherwise. So much of clutter accumulation goes back to fear. In this case, she feared being considered a "bad mom" because she equated holding on to his artwork with holding on to him. That kind of clutter association represents guilt and a skewed definition of your valuable role as a parent. You are actually doing your children a disservice if you hold on to everything that they scribble, paste, and color. You are imposing your own fears and guilt onto your children and are holding them back from healthy, emotional growth. You can forge an even closer and more meaningful bond with your children by practicing material detachment of stuff within your role as parent. The same rule holds true if you spoil your child with things. Things do not equal love. Again, stuff should never define you on any level.

One mother once told me, "When my daughter comes home with a party goody bag filled with all those little plastic toys and bad candy, I throw it all out after she goes to bed. She never even asks for it the next day!" At the time, when I heard this proclamation, I remember thinking in awe, "Wow, that sounds effective—yet extreme!" When in the same situation months later, holding a goody bag of bad candy and plastic junk, I tried it out. It worked without a hitch. Kids naturally amass an enormous amount of things and often don't even remember half of what they bring in when a little time passes. Their accumulation energy is as immense as their growing spirits! It's important to keep it in check or it can easily get out of control and take on monster energy of its own. It doesn't mean tossing *all* their possessions when the tots are sleeping. However, it does require keeping a vigilant handle on it all by having a focused system in place that you stick to. This will help them have an environment with a higher vibrational energy.

Holistic Home Kid Tips

- Either frame and display the best of your child's artwork or scan and archive it. You can even take a digital photo of it with your phone. Remaining artwork can be given or mailed to grandparents or other family members to enjoy or hung on the refrigerator for a week maximum, then dispersed or tossed.
- Have a designated place for everything—from a reachable hook for their backpacks and coats to a file folder mounted on the inside of a pantry door for their homework and school announcements. This sounds obvious, but if you don't have a system in place, keeping organized will feel fruitless.

- Get them involved, either by creating a habit of having them put their own items away or de-cluttering their own space. Make it fun and let them know that for everything that comes in, one thing has to come out.
- Be diligent with removing the toys that are no longer played with. If it's tough for your child to let go of some old toys, let them know how much other children in need will use and love the items they no longer use. If they still protest, put the toys in question in a box that's tucked away and make an agreement that if they still want them one month from now, they can have it back for a trial period. Chances are, they will not remember them.

THE MANY SCHOOLS OF FENG SHUI

Being that Feng Shui has been around for thousands of years, there have been dozens of interpretations—which are known as "schools"—over the centuries. Every school has its own value and richness, and nearly all have in common the main principles of obtaining health, wealth, and happiness. However, each one can conflict with the others in different ways, so I recommend picking one school you resonate with and sticking with that until you want to expand to others.

Early on, ancient Chinese farmers learned that by harnessing the forces of wind and water (the literal meaning of *Feng Shui*), they could have prolific crops, which also meant health and wealth. With wellness and prosperity in place, usually happiness would come next.

I have been trained in Black Hat Tantric Buddhist Feng Shui (BTB) founded by His Holiness Professor Lin Yun, who passed away in August 2010. Also known as Black Sect BTB, it places importance on the front door as the main conduit for beneficial chi yet also factors in modern psychology, urban planning, science, and interior design. Since there are so many schools of Feng Shui, it can get confusing. The table on the next page breaks down their basic differences.

Type of School of Feng Shui	Based Upon	Other Information
Land Form	Uses shapes in landscapes to determine auspicious positioning.	Mountains and water and their energies play a critical role in selecting sites of importance such as burial sites and business locations.
Compass	Emphasis is on direction: north, south, east, and west.	Uses a luopan (a tool that is like a complicated compass) along with factoring in your birth time and date to determine the best direction for you.
Flying Star	Uses dates of birth as essential information for determining positioning.	Examines the astrology of a building.
Pyramid	Modernizes old-word teachings.	Also known as the Western School of Feng Shui.
Four Pillars	Uses birth time, date, and place to create a natal chart.	Connects animal archetypes and elements to birth chi.
Eight Mansions	Divides the house into nine sections: the center, four most auspicious, and four least auspicious areas for certain activities for the occupants.	Also known as Eight House Feng Shui.
Classical	Blends both Form and Compass.	Most widely practiced worldwide.
Black Hat Sect Tantric Buddhism (BTB)	BTB has its roots from China, India, and Tibet. Influenced by Indian Buddhism.	Feng Shui map, called the bagua, can be superimposed on a site, floor plan, or room based on entryway.

THE FENG SHUI MAP

Over the past ten years of actively applying the Feng Shui map (or Bagua map) into my clients' homes, this is one concept that I have not updated, added to, or modified. It stands on its own, has always held true to modern-day needs, and has never failed to make the direct connections from the home to the life of the occupants. This energetic map will be used to determine where life areas correspond to your space, and you will discover how the correlations from the map to your own space can be extraordinary. You can mentally superimpose this map on any living space. The space of analysis can be an individual room, your entire floor plan, or the lot of land. The way you situate the map is to first locate your entrance. Next, superimpose the map on top of that space by lining up the entrance to the entryway wall side of the map. Your entrance can only be lined up with knowledge, career, or helpful people/travel. As you enter another floor of your home, the map needs to be lined up according to the entrance of that floor. Therefore, the way the map lines up on one floor may be different from another.

The map (shown in full on the next page) is divided into nine sections, called *guas*, and each gua is associated with a life area, color, and body part. Some guas are also associated with a body organ, season, and element. The nine sections represent the forces that control life and their fundamental nature, which have been derived from the ancient book of Chinese philosophy called *The I Ching*. One thing I had found frustrating in my Feng Shui studies is that it is rarely explained *why* this map is laid out the way it is. Most Feng Shui books have no explanation as to why it is positioned that way.

I recall one consultation where the husband walked into the room where I was sitting with his wife. He was a well-known CEO, highly intelligent and pragmatic. He was curious about what we were doing, and after his wife tried to explain a few concepts, he said, "I have one question. What determines the placement of wealth being here on the map and career being here and so forth?" I loved the question. It's rarely discussed and even renowned practitioners just take the map without question. It's important to question the process to understand it better. Once a practical explanation is offered, I find, it is easier to have faith in the process.

Here is what I have come up with: renditions of this map go back to ancient times, and there are only theories as to why exactly each section is laid out in the way it is. Many years ago, I was in a Feng Shui seminar led by British Feng Shui architect Benjamin Huntington when he shared his theory. This one made the most sense to me, and it stuck. He suggested that this map connects to our own primordial instincts, which have been deeply ingrained into our psyche for centuries. The hypothesis is that prehistoric man innately desired to store their goods or valuables in the farthest corner of their cave dwellings, which ended up becoming what is known today as the wealth gua. Tools for hunting and gathering were kept close to the front door in either the helpful people/travel gua or in knowledge/spirituality. Health issues took center focus. Then, family came together sharing knowledge and wealth, which placed them right between those two sections, and relationships naturally congregated toward the rear right, seeking a bit of privacy. Remaining guas sorted themselves out along the way. Here we are, thousands of years later, and most of these primordial concepts regarding our inherent placement feel natural, have stood the test of time, and are still applicable.

Looking at how these life areas correspond to your physical space, you can address where to take action to start the transformations you desire.

FENG SHUI BAGUA MAP

Align the door of either your entire floor plan or just a room to the entry way wall side of the bagua. Your door should line up to knowledge or career or helpful people/travel.

Wealth	Fame fire	Relationships
Family wood	Health earth	Creativity & Children metal
Knowledge & Spirituality	Career water	Travel & Helpful People

Entryway wall

BAGUA DESCRIPTIONS

Family

The middle portion on the left side relates to family, elders, and community. The element that has a natural position in this location is Wood and the corresponding color is green. The connecting organs are liver and gallbladder, and the body part is feet. (In addition to colors, shapes, and organs, there are certain parts of the body that connect to each gua. When you have an issue with that particular body part, it can be helpful to look to see where the corresponding gua is in your home and make adjustments accordingly.) This section governs new beginnings.

Wealth

On the far left corner lives the section that connects to abundance in all its forms: success, money, and prosperity. The corresponding color is purple, and the body part is the hips.

Health

Found in the center, the health area resonates to the color yellow and the element Earth. It relates to all issues concerned with stability and well-being. The connecting organs are the spleen, pancreas, and stomach.

Helpful People & Travel

All the people who make your life easier, protect or aid you throughout your lifetime, are all connected to this section. These may be friends, lawyers, mentors, teachers, doctors, caregivers, assistants, and angels. All forms of travel, either for business or pleasure, are connected to this space in the front right side. The connecting color is gray, and the body part is the head.

Children & Creativity

In the middle right side dwells the section that connects to completing new projects, imaginative resources, and children. The element Metal and the color white connect to this area. The body part is the mouth, and the connecting organs are lungs and large intestine.

Knowledge & Spirituality

Our inner journey of self-actualization, self-improvement, and spirituality reside here. This section, located in the front far left, connects to the color blue. The body part associated with this area is the hands.

Fame

The farthest middle section relates to our reputation, integrity, accomplishments, how we want the world to see us, and getting the recognition we deserve. It resonates to the element Fire and the color red. Eyes correspond to this section, and the connecting organs are the heart and small intestine.

Career

The middle front section connects to our vocational path, reflecting upon a situation and learning ability. Our vocation can be a paid occupational path, pastime, or a calling in life. It resonates to the color black and the element Water. The connecting body part is ears, and the related organ is the kidney.

Relationship

The farthest section on the upper right side relates to marriage and partnerships. The corresponding color is pink, and the connecting body part is the abdomen.

The bagua can be applied to any space, such as a room, an entire floor, a land lot, an entire city, hands, or face. You can even superimpose it onto your desktop. On the next page are examples of many different ways you can superimpose this Feng Shui tool in your surroundings.

You can superimpose the bagua map on a lot of land:

Wealth	Fame	Relationships
Family	Health	Children
Knowledge & Spirituality	Career	Helpful People & Travel

1   2   3

Superimpose the Feng Shui bagua map onto your property.
Always align the grid so that the entrance to your lot is lined up with either section 1, 2, or 3.

You can superimpose the bagua map on each floor of your house:

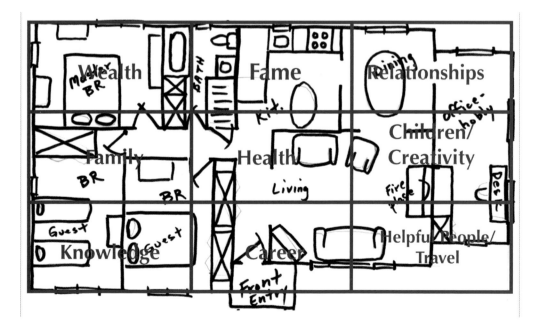

You can superimpose the bagua map on just one room:

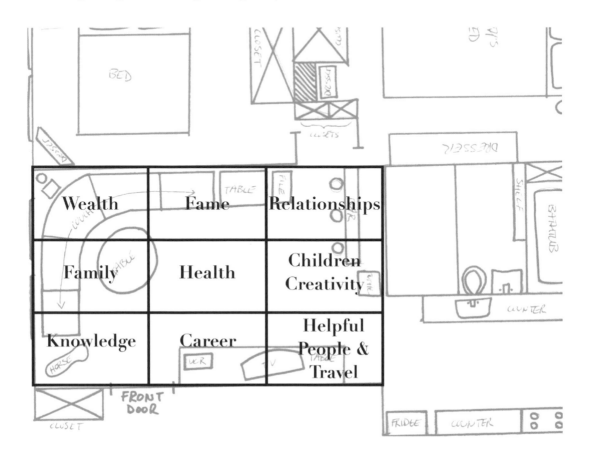

ADDRESSING THE MULTIPLE WAYS TO PLACE THE BAGUA

The first placement of the bagua should be on your entire floor plan. Think of this as the foundation for your Feng Shui guas. Each additional bagua placement (your lot, individual rooms) provides extra layers of ways to enhance particular guas. For example, if you are adjusting your wealth, it is best to look at all ways the wealth gua is situated in your environment and make adjustments in multiple areas. The bagua map can even be superimposed on a country, city, or community. For country placement, use the airport or harbor with the most inbound and outbound flow of traffic as the mouth of chi. To place it on a city, use the airport or highway with the greatest flow of traffic as the main entrance.

TROUBLESHOOTING

If two doors to a space are used equally, determine which one is predominately used. If that is still ambiguous, go with the door that is *structurally* designated as the main door. Even if you use your back door every day as your front door, align the bagua map with the front door.

For each floor, you can determine the mouth of chi separately by locating the entrance to that individual floor. If you have a shape that is not rectangular, the basic rule to determine if a section is missing or strengthened is by determining the proportion to the other sections.

The floor plan below is an example of an extension in the fame gua.

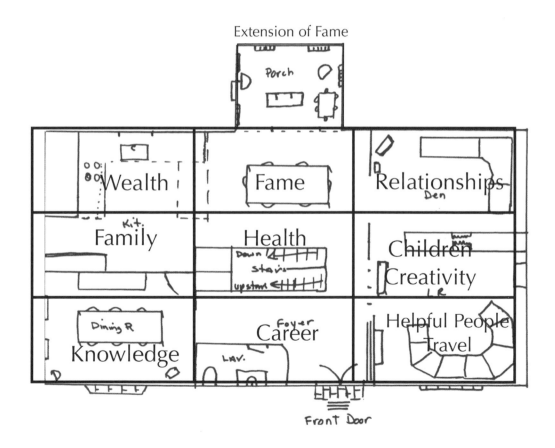

Extension of Fame

Below is a home with the entire wealth gua missing as well as some portions of fame, family, and relationship. When a missing area is smaller than one gua, like the fame gua in the floor plan above, it becomes an extension.

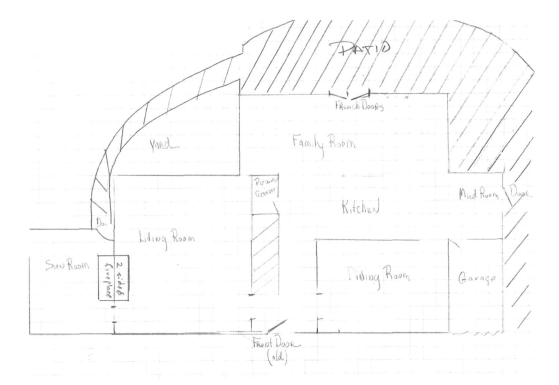

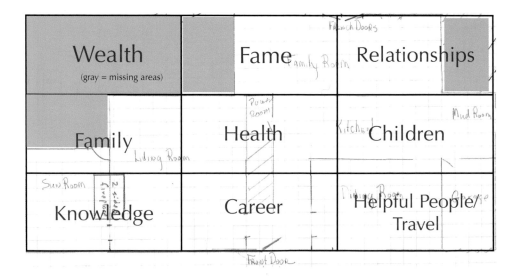

Holistic Spirit Tip

You are a mirror for your environment and vice versa. Every area of your life (wealth, health, relationships, career, family, etc.) is related energetically to your living space. When the chi cannot flow freely throughout your home, you are creating the propensity for similar sluggishness and inactivity in the area of your life that connects to the bagua.

THE SPIRIT AND CLUTTER

Harnessing the spiritual energies of nature to create a safe, protected, and thriving home is a notion that has been around for thousands of years. This concept is a primordial instinct programmed deep within our souls. Global concerns, technological dependence, energy depletion, financial instability, and busier, stress-filled lives have affected our day-to-day living. Being bombarded with boundless stimuli and countless consumer goods have added more clutter to our spirit and changed the way we dwell. All the clutter that surrounds you in your home is energetically connected to you. If you have lots of it, it's dragging you down and draining your spirit. Often, the more clutter you have, the more disconnected you are to your spirituality. When you have thinned out your possessions and kept only the things that are sacred to you, you can easily live a more meaningful, consecrated, and thoughtful life.

Many people view success as having lots of luxury items and identify their own self-worth, accomplishments, or ego with these things. But it's not how massive your house is, and it's not how large your engagement ring is. We all know that money can't buy you happiness, and we've heard the saying so many times it's become trite. But truly, if desire for things is what is driving you, you will never be truly happy. The initial post-purchase glee will fade fast, and the emptiness of what else you don't have will expand to a deeper abyss in your spiritual psyche. Understand your motives for wanting more.

I'm not saying you should be living a monk-like existence. Manifesting abundance in the form of prosperity can provide a great deal of freedom and peace of mind. Be clear in your motives and pure in your mantras and visualizations, and focus on nourishing your spirit. Try to teach the children you know to value quality time together over things and to be grateful for what they already have.

If need be, redefine your idea about what success is. Instead of success equaling more and more things, try letting success equal love or being able to spend quality time with your family. Add to your definition of success by how you can help others thrive. And remember, when you help or give to others and you feel the need to herald your altruistic deeds or make a big deal of the gifts you give, it diminishes the spiritual meaning of your intentions. Don't give for validation or recognition.

Don't keep asking the receiver if they love the gift you gave them. Next time you help someone out and you notice that, for example, you are tweeting a picture of yourself at the food bank dishing soup, ask yourself, "Am I looking for approval or admiration from others by sharing this? Would I still be doing this if no one knew about it? What is driving me right now?" If you give for the sake of creating an altruistic persona, it will backfire. Part of spiritual de-cluttering means releasing your expectations that are associated with the stuff that surrounds you and identifying the real reasons you give to others and the spiritual connections to the actual physical stuff in your home.

SPIRITUAL CLUTTER AND THE BAGUA

The Feng Shui map, the bagua, can help you determine the spiritual meanings behind your clutter.

Wealth

Clutter in this area clogs up the flow of prosperity and impedes you from receiving plenty of opportunities in your life. Increasing finances can be very difficult when the wealth area is in disarray or loaded with clutter.

Fame

Disorder in this area can cause your reputation to weaken. You can lose passion and drive if this gua gets out of order. If you want to improve how others see you, make sure this area is neat and organized. If you want to improve your reputation, keep everything sparkly and shiny here.

Relationships

When this area is disorganized, it becomes difficult to sustain healthy relationships or attract new ones. If you are in a relationship or looking to bring in a new one, make sure this area is not loaded with items from your past or contains broken objects. Make sure this section does not have stagnant energy—otherwise, you will draw more of that stagnation into your relationships. A cluttered relationship gua is like getting involved with someone who has a ton of baggage. We all have some, but let yours be a small, manageable carry-on, not a job for a full-time bellhop.

Family

Disorganization in this gua can cause problems with authority figures, parents, family members, or community. Clean this area to support shining relations with relatives and neighbors.

Health

When the center of your space is in need of order, it can significantly affect your health and general well-being. This is the least common area to accumulate clutter, since most of it finds its way to the periphery of a space. So, if this is where your disorganization dwells, be fastidious in creating a new vision.

Children & Creativity

If this area has stuck energy, count on delays in finishing projects and blocks in creativity. Relationships with children will suffer if this area is cluttered.

Knowledge & Spirituality

Personal growth and the ability to see oneself clearly and to make wise choices can be hindered when clutter accumulates in this gua.

Career

Your vocational path will feel like an uphill struggle if this gua is loaded with energy blocks. If your professional goals are unclear, check if this area is messy.

Helpful People & Travel

Disorganization and clutter in this area can block the flow of support in your life. If you feel like you are alone or are not getting the breaks you deserve, make sure this gua is as tidy as possible. If you are having trouble traveling or moving, clean this area even if you feel like it already appears orderly.

HOW TO SPIRITUALLY DE-CLUTTER

Now that everything has a place, you have de-cluttered your mind and home, and you have identified the spiritual connections, it's time to cleanse the invisible mess— spiritual clutter. Spiritual clutter is the predecessor energy of your home as well as the current energy that is imbued in the energetic atmosphere of your surroundings. Often you can pick up on the energy of the people who lived there before you. If they had particular and persistent troubles while living there, you might have similar ones. Even if there were no bad occurrences or you are living in a brand new home, it's still important to clean the energetic clutter in the air. Residual energy from all the people involved in the building process may still linger.

You can clean the leftover energy by performing a clearing ceremony. This is one of my favorite things to do because, afterward, spaces just *feel* different. You know the feeling you get when your home is freshly cleaned? Well, this is similar, except it's a cleaning of the leftover energy of a space.

This is not some New Age hocus-pocus; clearing ceremonies have been around for thousands of years in China, Tibet, India, and Greece. Even today, Catholic churches use them when wafting frankincense around to symbolically cleanse and purify surroundings. Native Americans performed cleansing rituals regularly with sage, which is the most popular cleansing tool for Feng Shui consultants today and

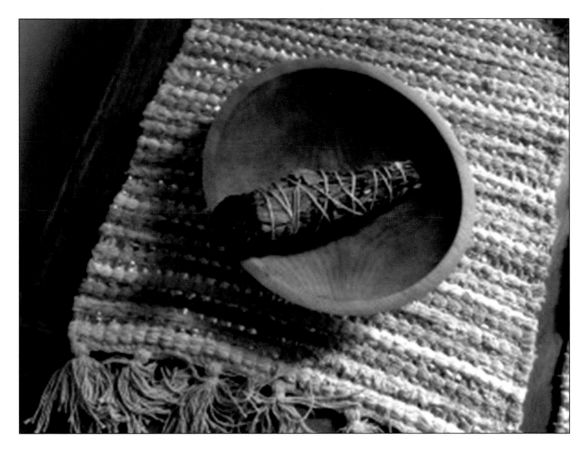

is what I highly recommend you use. Over the years, one of the rituals I've stopped using involved cinnabar. Many Feng Shui experts still sprinkle it around clients' homes because they believe it expels negativity. Originally from volcanoes and bright red in color, it was believed to be magic powder centuries ago. I believe that bringing mercury sulfide inside your home is never safe. It can be fatal—especially to children and animals—if inhaled, ingested, or touched by skin. Stick to burning a bundle of sweat grass, palo santo, or sage. They are equally powerful and nontoxic.

Conduct a Clearing Ceremony

The predominant energy that occurs in a home over time becomes imbued in the atmosphere of that space. It's what makes some homes "feel" different from others for no explicable reason. Whether it is mostly illness and anger or love and laughter, your home's atmosphere will take on that energy. The goal is to set up your home to support the inevitable ups and downs of life and be able to shed the negative layers before they pile on in your space. The simplest yet most effective remedy is to air out your home for at least five minutes every day and allow as much natural light as possible to filter in. The best way to scrub the air clean of lingering energy is to burn some sage to energetically clean the atmosphere on a deeper level.

Start by opening all your windows and turning on all your lights. If possible, put on lively, upbeat music. Center yourself and connect to the spiritual or religious figure of your choice or a loved one who has passed on.

Light some incense, sweat grass, or sage, and walk through your home while wafting the smoke around. These dried herb bundles have become so mainstream now, you can find them at virtually all of your local, organic, whole food stores. (Be sure to hold a bowl under the burning herbs so that you can catch any stray embers.) If you have bells, chimes, or gongs, add them into the mix to elevate the sound component. Recite your favorite chants or prayers, or just simply state out loud what you are cleaning out. "I am clearing away all the bad mojo in the kitchen from the terrible fight I had last night with my husband!" Or what you no longer want in your life. "I am clearing out all the toxic people in my life!" Or, clear away a lingering feeling. "I am clearing out feeling afraid" or "I am clearing out the energy from those who have lived here before me." Concentrate on cleaning the air from previous arguments, sad events, misfortune, illness, or bad luck.

As you walk through your home, visualize you are cleansing any negative patterns and you are strengthening positive ones. You can call in a loved one who has passed, your guardian angel, God, or any deity you connect with. What's important is to connect the energy of your home and your intentions going forward. Pay particular attention to where clutter formerly resided the most. Visualize that everything has a place and your surroundings will continue to remain clean and organized. Finish the process by giving gratitude for your space. Imagine the entire home filled with a bright, golden light. Thank it for containing your life. This can truly be a highly effective method in taking your cleansing to another level of intensity by consecrating the energies in your space and affirming your objectives.

De-cluttering your mind, body, spirit, and home is vital in living life more fully. It is easier to feel joy, think with clarity, and make your goals happen. By applying holistic principles in new ways that go beyond just moving your stuff, you can truly begin to create an environment that is balanced, harmonious, and congruent with your life goals. With a holistic mind, body, and spirit, you are now clear, strong, and focused, and ready to begin the process of seeing and connecting with your space—and yourself—differently. Let's move on to your health, your goals, and the timing of it all.

CHAPTER THREE

Get in Your Groove: Taking Cues from Nature

"The goal of life is living in agreement with nature."

—Zeno (335 BC–264 BC)

When I did a consultation on a massive Manhattan home, not a bed, desk, or stove was improperly positioned. There was an entire household management staff that oversaw every aspect of domestic operations. Clutter was virtually nonexistent, colors were right on, and chi was mostly flowing in a graceful, undulating way. The residence showcased rare building materials from exotic locations that were constructed in extraordinary ways. A world-famous architect designed the focal point staircase. Every day a floral designer on staff tended to each petal on display. The home was a magical showplace with seldom seen design details, high-tech gadgetry, and lush opulence everywhere you looked. Everything on the surface looked perfect.

You might be sensing that a "but" is on its way. Insert it here. The word *conflict* was present in excess throughout the homeowner's language during the entire consultation. I soon discovered the source of all this conflict resided in the tormented heart of Lynn, the woman who called this place home. Lynn had manifested her inner conflict throughout her home in the most widespread and surest way this disruptive force can come to the surface—through nature. Nature *inside* your home, you might be asking? Yes, indeed. And it shows up in a boatload of ways. If you are feeling disconnected, conflicted, out of sorts, or out of sync, chances are the ways that nature is expressed—or not—in your home is having a big impact on these feelings. The first way we will examine how nature is expressed in your home is through the Five Elements. Fire, Water, Metal, Earth, and Wood are one of the most expressive conduits for conflict in your environment.

Conflict is an imbalance of energy and the antithesis of a harmonious space. The more it shows up in your life in various ways, such as through an illness, stress, or recurring challenges, the more closely the five-elemental flow of balance and harmony need to be examined throughout the home. Since human beings and nature share similar universal forces and cycles, it is logical that certain aspects of nature can act as a guide for a variety of human conditions. If two opposing elements are competing with one another, then conflict can arise. If one element is dominating the home or is conspicuously not present, an imbalance may occur.

During Lynn's initial walk-through of the home, I asked various questions: "Would you tell me about this artwork? Do you and your husband sleep well? How does this home represent you?"

I felt as if the very essence of conflict was imbued in the energetic foundation of the home with every story of construction and design, embedded with personality clashes each step of the way. Lynn informed me that conflict began during the massive renovations before move-in ("The contractors and architects were in constant conflict during the entire time"). Conflict even surrounded two pictures hung side by side ("The artists are in personal conflict with each other and were not pleased that we hung their work next to one another"). Conflict was present in the interior design process ("There was terrible conflict between myself and the interior designer"). Conflict was present in some relationships in the house ("I have had a great deal of conflict with my household manager"). Midway though our consultation, I touched upon the source of Lynn's conflict: living what she called a "privileged lifestyle" while feeling guilty for doing so. Lynn was private yet open to the process of having a stranger in her heavily secured home as she candidly answered my intimate questions. It concerned me that conflict plagued her so exhaustively. Nearly every answer she gave me mentioned the word *conflict*. It hovered in the home with an ominous presence.

The one element nearly void in their home was Wood. The one place it existed was where Lynn liked to retreat for some solace—to a hand-carved Japanese soaking tub made of teak. (Although when she showed me the tub, she said she was "conflicted about keeping it because its upkeep is so high-maintenance".) There was an extreme abundance of metal throughout the home, from appliances to grand staircases to stone flooring and light fixtures. In the Five Element Theory (see diagram on the next page), Fire controls Metal. I suggested adding more Wood and Water. Water feeds Wood (think of water nourishing trees). The addition of more Wood would buffer the excess of metal. The color green (which represents the element Wood) was an absent color that, when added, would help bring it all together. Adding more plants inside their home would add the Wood life force that felt lacking in such an otherwise beautiful home.

The main gist here is that, in nature, there is a particular way that these forces reside together that will either be supportive to one another or not. When these fundamental elements are out of balance in your home, you are going to be affected by it in some way.

Understanding the Five Elements is the key to harmony in your environment and in yourself. The Five Element Theory is derived from Taoism. This component of Taoism relates to living in harmony and balance with the cycles of nature. Water, Wood, Fire, Earth, and Metal are the essential and omnipotent energies that can potentially create or destroy the energetic balances in our environment. Their effects in our lives are profound. Intentionally tapping into their energies can instigate change and transformation. Each element has special associations with particular areas of life, certain emotions, personality traits, shapes, colors, seasons, and also with particular organs in the human body.

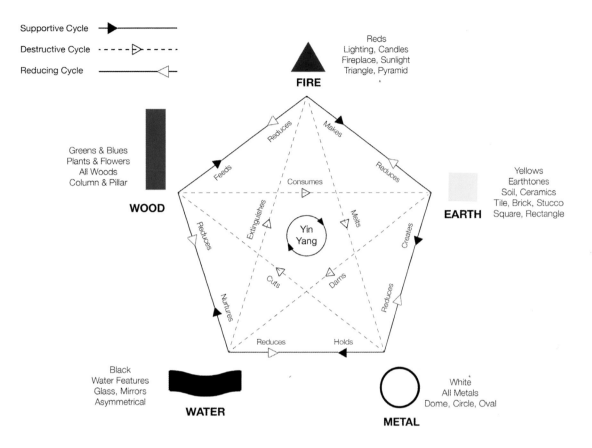

The study of the Five Elements is an early form of science that the Chinese started thousands of years ago by living close to the soil and recognizing the connections between themselves and the Earth's rhythms. They realized three main points:

- Humankind energetically vibrates in tandem with nature.
- We are constantly in a state of flux from birth to death.
- We are interconnected with the Universe.

These philosophies spawned the antediluvian book *I Ching*, which presents the metaphysics of Chinese culture to help explain past, current, and future events. The

I Ching led to Taoism, which views the Universe and its accomplishments as being cyclical, transformative, and interactive. The Tao (pronounced *dow*) reflects the eternal rhythm of the Universe and the way of man within it. Examples of the cyclical ways nature surrounds us range from massive scales of planetary cycles down to a woman's fertility cycle. From the life cycle of birth to death, *everything* is connected through constant cycles that operate interdependently.

Quantum physicist John Stewart Bell said, "No theory of reality compatible with quantum theory can require spatially separate events to be independent." I know this may sound abstract, so here is the simplified version: *We are all connected with each other and with nature. We operate in interrelated cycles that affect one another.* Furthermore, when we harness the cyclical power of nature, we can live better—more effortlessly. We can make smoother transitions to readily accept the bumps along the way. We are aligned for opportunities and are more easily able to instigate the changes we want to see. Also, when at our optimal Universal flow, we are supporting our higher self and reaching our greatest potential. It is one of life's secrets, yet it's all around us, from sunup to sundown. Pay attention to the cues, cycles, and interconnectedness of the world around you, and you'll begin to make the connections too.

The Five Elements have a natural cyclical flow together. As with any cycle in life, the flow of transformation can be clockwise or counterclockwise. This flow can be established by how the elements wind up being present (or not) in our environment and how they are purposely situated (or not). When flowing clockwise, it is described as the supportive cycle. Each element is assisting the other, enabling an effortless flow from one transition to the other. When counterclockwise, it is described as the reducing cycle because each element has the potential to control the next.

A supportive cycle is depicted as Wood fueling Fire; Fire then creates Earth (ash); Earth then produces Metal (minerals); Metal attracts Water (condensation); Water then nourishes Wood. On the other hand, a destructive cycle is one where Wood consumes Earth (absorbing its nutrients); Earth dams Water (turning it into mud); Water extinguishes Fire; Fire melts Metal; and Metal destroys Wood

(Metal blades cut Wood). How this translates to your environment could mean an unknowingly misplaced water feature could be smoldering the flames of your love life.

Just because the supportive cycle means generating or creating does not mean that the destructive cycle is a pejorative flow. The destructive cycle can be used positively to prevent excess development, keep other elements in check, and maintain balance. When following the dotted line of its course and seeing how, for example, Water puts out Fire—the element to mitigate that would be Wood.

All elements should be present throughout the home more or less equally according to your emotional and physical needs. If you are not in tune with your imbalances—such as an unknown illness or a behavior you are not aware of—try looking at the surface levels of your surroundings for clues.

FEELING IMBALANCED? LOOK IN YOUR ENVIRONMENT

Think of the essence of each element and their properties. For example, the color for Fire is red, which is a Yang color, and among other stimulating properties can promote proliferation, aggression, and production. It is not recommended for those with cancer because it is too active a color for cells that are already rapidly growing and mutating. However, those suffering from lethargy might find the color red brings joy and motivation and would fare well with a more substantial amount of this element present. Take note of the omnipresent elements in your home, and ask yourself: is this excess enabling or controlling an imbalance in my life? For example, if you are surrounded by a great deal of water—a bay in your backyard, water imagery in all your artwork, water fountains, and aquariums—and you have a tendency to be overemotional, all of this water could potentially enhance this tendency even more. There are situations, however, when an occupant purposely chooses environmental embellishments that bring about the change they subconsciously desire. Let's say you are surrounded by all the same water imagery, are not empathetic, live mostly in your head, are consumed by work—yet you have an awareness of your shortcomings and a deep desire to change them, or at the very least, you know that Water offers you a balance in your life. It is a possibility that your higher self brought in what was needed. Although this scenario is not as common as the first, it is often present in those who are beginning to develop their sense of self-awareness or are on the verge of their own personal transformation. Throughout your life, you may have been drawn to certain elements unknowingly that served a purpose for what you subconsciously needed at the time. You may have loved yellow as a child but barely use it as an adult. You will discover that the elements you are drawn to or avoid will reveal a lot about yourself. If you already have a known issue, think of the corresponding element as you go through the following questions.

DO YOU TEND TO AVOID USING PARTICULAR ELEMENTS?

Carefully examine what colors, shapes, or actual elements you are apt to avoid or choose less of in your environment. Once that is established, discover what that element represents and honestly assess whether those properties can benefit you. A person who is lacking enthusiasm and incentive might be surrounding themselves in a safe nest of pastels. Adding the Fire element can be the driving force that is needed. Conversely, those who have a tendency toward aggressive or volatile behavior should avoid excess use of the color red and the element Fire.

DO YOU FEEL MORE COMFORTABLE AROUND SOME ELEMENTS MORE THAN OTHERS?

If you are aligning yourself with particular elements, it may be out of comfort, or possibly you are tapping into certain characteristics of that element that you are in need of. Usually we choose to surround ourselves with the element that we feel most at ease around. It is human nature to want to avoid what makes us feel uncomfortable, but nine times out of ten, it's by going to those places that we grow and transform the most.

HARNESSING THE ENERGIES OF NATURE, THEN AND NOW

In 4000 BC, the ancient Chinese used lunar, solar, and astronomy phases in conjunction with cues from creative and destructive elemental cycles for guidance in obtaining food, strength, and protection. The constant process of synchronizing with the natural rhythms of the world has guided the earliest cultures in many aspects of living, such as farming, medicine, and military. Now more than ever, we are drawing upon the workings of nature to build an awareness of the elements and how to use them to our benefit. New ways for developing renewable sources of energy are being found to harness the elemental power of the wind (chi), sun (Fire), and sea (Water) to live cleaner and greener lives. By living in ways that are utilizing and caring for the natural resources of the planet, you are syncopating your own natural rhythms toward a holistically balanced life.

MY STORY: THE NEXT CYCLE

Every six weeks, I am supposed to go to my hematologist/oncologist for a blood test and checkup. This is not an event that I particularly look forward to, and I often extend the time in between by an extra month or so. It starts off in the waiting room, sitting elbow-to-elbow for several hours among patients who, by sight, appear far worse off than me; skeletal frames wearing particle or oxygen masks, looking scared and hopeless. It usually ends with the doctor palpating my spleen, reviewing my blood values, and then me needing to get a phlebotomy to get rid of all the extra blood my bone marrow is proliferating. Sometimes, if my favorite nurse is not around, there are big challenges in getting a good vein. This part can make me panic. But I am very lucky. For the most part, in over fourteen years since I was diagnosed, this has been my basic protocol of Western treatment.

One day I started to feel my enlarged spleen even more than usual. It got to the point where I could only wear tent-like dresses, had trouble finding a good position to sleep in, and would feel very uncomfortable when I touched that area. I asked my hem/onc if my spleen would ever be able to shrink from being so enlarged. He told me no. I told him, "You just watch. I'm going to shrink it."

I had gone to many acupuncturists over the years. It was only when I met Rebecca Tracey that I felt I found my mighty, humble healer extraordinaire. I had been going to her occasionally over the last two years, but now with my spleen becoming a pressing matter, I wanted to kick it up a notch and go weekly. I randomly chose 10 a.m. appointments. Within only two weeks, I started to feel a significant difference for the better. Before each session, I would also try to dovetail a holistic adjustment in my home that focused on the element Earth, which connects to the spleen. Sometimes it was simply making sure that I had absolutely no clutter in the Earth gua (center) of my home.

While in the midst of writing this chapter, I went to my regularly scheduled appointment with Rebecca, and we talked about the Five Elements Theory. She told me about another component of this system, the Organ Clock Theory, where each of the twelve organs has a particular time of day when it functions at its prime. "The Dalai Lama gets up between 3 a.m. and 5 a.m. to chant, because that is the best time for the lungs. Then the next cycle, 5 a.m. to 7 a.m., is optimal for the large intestine for elimination. Next, he will eat because 7 a.m. to 9 a.m. is the time for the stomach," she explained. The next cycle, 9 a.m. to 11 a.m., is the optimal functioning time for the spleen. I had unintentionally made my one-hour acupuncture appointments at 10 a.m. Often, when we are in sync with our Universal energy, we unknowingly make choices that are in alignment with that natural flow. You watch—you will, too!

Organ Clock Theory

3 a.m.–5 a.m.	Lungs
5 a.m.–7 a.m.	Large Intestine
7 a.m.–9 a.m.	Stomach
9 a.m.–11 a.m.	Spleen

11 a.m.–1 p.m.	Heart
1 p.m.–3 p.m.	Small Intestine
3 p.m.–5 p.m.	Urinary Bladder
5 p.m.–7 p.m.	Kidney
7 p.m.–9 p.m.	Pericardium
9 p.m.–11 p.m.	Endocrine System
11 p.m.–1 a.m.	Gallbladder
1 a.m.–3 a.m.	Liver

My spleen was feeling smaller, and all was going well until Rebecca took an extended maternity leave, and I was left without acupuncture treatments for nine months. I was hesitant to start anew with someone else, so I just waited until she returned. Six months into this gap, my doctor informed me that my spleen had grown two centimeters. When Rebecca returned, I resumed my weekly appointments, and six months later, in June 2013, my doctor was shocked and pleased to report that my spleen was now significantly smaller. "I think it's the acupuncture," he said. "Keep doing what you are doing." In the same way that acupuncture harnesses, tweaks, and adjusts the energetic pathways that flow throughout your body, the adjustments and changes that you are learning to make throughout this book are similarly working with the energy in your home and, in turn, within yourself. When aiming to optimize your health, the more you can holistically merge together your thinking, timing, energetic adjustments, and physical changes in your environment, the greater your results can be.

The Five Element Theory has been a part of Eastern medicine since tenth century BC, which is a long time to be tried and tested. The sequence of the five phases can describe interactions, transformations, and relationships in nature and in Man. Medical philosophers used this dynamic cycle of change to explain and treat disease for thousands of years. Recently, the *Washington Post* reported that a growing number of traditionally trained physicians are now incorporating acupuncture, Reiki, and herbs into their protocol. These traditional Chinese medicine–based approaches are all a result of the Five Element Theory, which is now frequently being implemented to treat mental, spiritual, and physical imbalances.

THE BODY AND THE FIVE ELEMENTS

Of all nature's phenomena, the human body is perhaps the most miraculous. We are made of multiple complex and interconnected systems, such as the skeletal, muscular, digestive, nervous, lymphatic, cardiovascular, reproductive, and more, which are all striving for harmony and balance. When the human body falls out of balance, the result is disease. The Five Element Theory in Chinese medicine correlates different organs and bodily systems to the nature of each particular element. When out of balance, you will most likely see how this element is represented in your home.

Fire

Cardiovascular functions, and any heart problems, are all connected to the element Fire. Symptoms such as high blood pressure, strokes, blocked arteries, blood diseases, and angina are related to the Fire network.

Water

Kidney and bladder as well as all fluid metabolism and elimination systems are related to the element Water. The kidney stores the essence of growth and regeneration, controlling teeth, bones, marrow, brain, and inner ear function.

Wood

Liver, adrenals, and gallbladder are connected to the element Wood. When there is an imbalance, gallstones, headaches, cramping, and impulsive behavior can ensue.

Metal

Lungs and colon are ruled by the element Metal. When a disparity occurs, colds, pneumonia, or asthma may occur. Colon and intestinal issues are connected to this element.

Earth

Stomach, spleen, and pancreas are connected to the element Earth. When this network is disturbed, indigestion, bloating, and fatigue can occur.

> **Holistic Body Tip: Take Your Medication with Your Cellular Cycles**
> Chronotherapy means coordinating your medical treatment with your body's natural biological rhythms to fight disease. Timing and dosages of medication are coordinated with the natural rhythms of the body for optimal health. Organs, blood flow, and heart activity all have certain rhythms that ebb and flow throughout the day. These cellular rhythms are in direct connection to nature and can vary according to seasonal cycles, menstrual cycles, sleep cycles, yearly cycles, or more. Your doctor might already be aware of basic fluctuations of biorhythms that your body presets in anticipation of daily activities, such as blood pressure being the highest midday and the lowest at bedtime. Hopefully your doctor will be open to helping you create a schedule of optimal times for your medical treatment that integrates known fluctuations and the Organ Clock Theory. Always confer with your doctor before changing any medication routines.

OPTIMIZING YOUR BODY

The Organ Clock Theory (page 64–65) has a circadian rhythm, which means it is repeated every twenty-four hours. Nature creates our biological clocks, which govern activity, rest, sleep, excretion, chemical composition, regulation of tissue fluids, and glands. Keep this timetable in mind to holistically adjust whatever internal organ you have a challenge with. In addition, make your energetic adjustments in the connecting gua of that particular organ. For example, if you have high blood pressure (a heart issue), make Fire adjustments in your Fame gua between 11 a.m. and 1 p.m. Assess how the connecting element is being represented in your home. Is it absent? Is it present in excess? Use your intuition to guide you.

If kidney stones, urinary tract infections, or water retention is a problem, look at how the element Water is represented in your environment. How is the plumbing working throughout your home? Between 3 p.m. and 7 p.m., repair any leaks, and assess if the bathroom (which represents water) is in need of maintenance. Is there a pool located at the home? Is it clean and working properly? Are there water features like ponds or fountains, and are they clean and working properly? Are there any drains inside or outside your property that are clogged or moving sluggishly? If you have liver, lung, or stomach ailments, just look at the corresponding time and element associated with that organ, and look around for anything that is out of balance, in need of repair, or missing, and adjust accordingly.

OVERVIEW OF THE FIVE ELEMENTS

The key to working with the Five Elements is first to be able to clearly identify them and become familiar with their expressions. They can be literally and symbolically represented by various stages and manifestations of that energy throughout your

The Five Element Table					
	Fire	**Water**	**Metal**	**Earth**	**Wood**
Color	Red	Black	Gray	Yellow	Green
Gua	Fame	Career	Helpful People	Health	Family
Found In	Lighting, Candles	Fountains, Pools, Streams	Metal, Cement, Rocks, Stainless Steel	Adobe, Brick, Tile, Ceramics	Wood Furniture, Plants
Shape	Triangles	Asymmetrical Shapes	Spheres, Domes	Rectangles	Pillars, Columns
Season	Summer	Winter	Autumn	Harvest	Spring
Body Part	Heart	Kidneys	Lungs	Stomach	Liver
Key Use	Aids with Change	Adaptability	Communication	Security	Motivation

home, body, emotions, and spirit. It takes close inspection in your surroundings and in yourself to observe the various levels of depiction of the corresponding elements.

CASE STUDY: MARGARET LUCE

The Five Elements can be present in the actual elements themselves or colors, shapes, symbolic representations, or fabrics. Homeowner Margaret Luce says of her home, "I've always collected great fabrics, mostly unappreciated vintage with beautiful textures, and then I dream of what should be on a settee, a modern armchair, a stool, etc. That's when the magic begins. I really think like a set designer, and I create different nooks that evolve into conversation pieces, to sit and enjoy. For example, I recently just refurbished a wonderful Queen Anne chair and covered it with my couture Versace dress alongside American made white Ultrasuede fabric for $9.99 a yard."

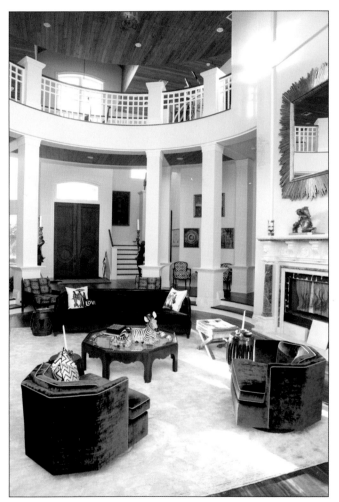

Margaret Luce's living room has a balance of all the five elements, both literally and symbolically.

Fire

The color red, triangular shapes, and actual fire such as fireplaces and the blaze from candles all demonstrate this element. The season is summer, and the emotion is joy.

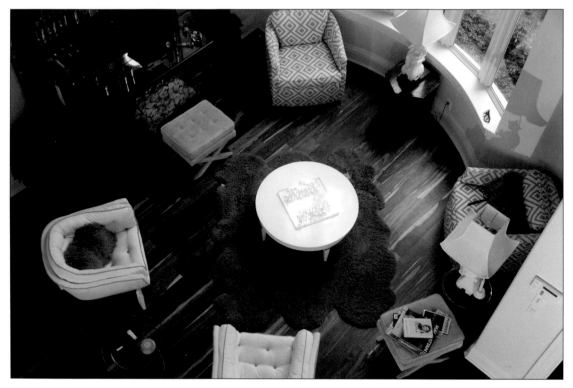

Luce says, "I'm always tempted to move things around or buy something with a pop of color to make my own. When I'm creating, it's important to me that it's authentic."

Water

Symbolized by the color black, asymmetrical shapes, and water features such as fountains, ponds, and reflective surfaces. The season is winter, and the emotion is fear.

Wood

The color green, and pillar and column shapes represent Wood, and representation can be found in wood furniture, plants, and plant-based materials. The season is spring, and the emotion is anger.

Earth

Yellow is the color representing Earth, and the square shapes depict it. The season is late summer, and the emotion is sympathy.

Metal

The color white, dome shapes, and metal materials (bronze, gold, silver, tin, copper, nickel, brass, and steel) as well as igneous rocks and minerals such as marble, granite, and cement represent the element Metal. The season is autumn, and the emotion is grief.

THE MIND AND THE FIVE ELEMENTS

Being that humans are cyclical microcosms that reflect some of the same patterns of nature, we can begin to understand the impact of the elements and their meanings within ourselves. Each one of us has the energy of all Five Elements within us, but with a propensity for one. When there are excessive or deficient expressions—either within our immediate environment or ourselves—we experience an imbalance in ways from emotional to personality conflicts to disease.

Excessive Water in an environment might lead the occupants to feel spacey, unfocused, and overly emotional. They can restrain those feelings by adding the element Earth to control the excessive Water. An abundance of Wood in your home might be adding to an atmosphere that fosters self-righteousness and inflexibility. Introduce balance by adding Metal. A deficit of the Fire element might be furthering sluggishness, and by simply adding more Fire, the energy of motivation becomes initiated in your surroundings.

REACHING YOUR GOALS WITH THE FIVE ELEMENTS

The Five Elements correspond to different natural locations in your home as well as specific areas of your life. Adding certain elements into your surroundings can assist you in creating a supportive environment for your goals. Refer to pages 43–44 to identify where each area corresponds to in your home.

If you are looking to **enhance your reputation and integrity**, add the Fire element into your life. Fire can be found in candles, lighting, triangular shapes, and the color red. Whether you are hanging artwork with red tones or lighting a candle, place this element in its natural location—the fame section—and visualize yourself getting the recognition you deserve.

If you are seeking **spirituality, inspiration, and relaxation**, welcome the element Water into your life. This element is found in water fountains, pools, fish tanks, and streams and is symbolized by asymmetrical shapes and the color black. Its natural location is in the career area of your home. A water fountain also promotes a healthy, refreshing release of negative ions, which provides a positive sense of well-being and makes breathing easier.

Looking to enhance your **communication, independence, and mental focus?** Bring Metal into your environment. This element is found in all metals, cement, rocks, and stainless steel and is symbolized by the color gray, and sphere and dome shapes. Envision improved communication as you add this element to its natural location in your home, the helpful people and travel area.

Intuition, creativity, expansion, and growth are all energetically fostered by the element Wood. Wood furniture, live plants, plant-based materials, the color green, and pillar shapes all represent this developing element. It is beneficial to have around children to aid in their growing spirits. Add Wood to your family section in your home, and imagine the rivers of creativity flowing your way.

Earth is the element that enhances **physical strength, boosts stability and practicality, and creates a nurturing environment for caregivers**. It can be found in earthenware, ceramics, tile, and adobe and is symbolized by rectangular shapes and the color yellow. Add your pottery and yellow colors to its corresponding natural location, the health section, and visualize the security that you need.

SYNC UP WITH THE SEASONS

Use seasonal cues to guide you when working on personal goals. Winter is a phase for reflection and stillness, so it's a good time for solo activities of contemplation like writing in a journal or learning to meditate. Fall is for harvesting, so utilize this energy to research, to assemble like minds for a project, or to gather your ideas and resources. Spring is a time of renewal and beginnings. Try to shed the old and negative by instigating healthy routines such as a detox or cleansing program, a juice fast, or a new exercise routine. Summer is a time of fullness and completion. Beget this energy in your life by often acknowledging what you are grateful for, paying forward good deeds, and completing projects.

Season	Best Time To . . .
Fall	Fall is a time of harvesting and gathering your ideas. Use this time to prepare yourself for future goals like researching for a book, collecting ideas for redecorating, or planning a wedding or trip.
Winter	Winter is a time of stillness and scarcity. Utilize this time for solo activities like starting a meditation practice, a bird watching hobby, or journaling.
Spring	Spring is a time for renewal and new beginnings. It's a great time to start a detox, clean out a closet, or begin a new workout routine. Think fresh action and new starts.
Summer	Summer is a time for expansion and playfulness. Make time for outdoor activities and tap into ways that bring joy into your life.

HARNESS THE CYCLES AROUND YOU

Ancient principles teach us that nature is in flux, yet cyclical. Humankind follows the same cyclical laws. You might already be bringing out seasonal decorations for the holidays or swapping out your warm weather clothes for your cold wardrobe. Take it a step further. Rotate your collectibles with the change of seasons. By revolving your chosen objects in accordance with the cycles of the environment, you can harmoniously shift the energy in your home to create a cohesive atmosphere as well as create the illusion of more space. Besides rotating your décor, try switching your furniture configurations around in accordance with the shift in seasons to subconsciously enhance your own sense of balance in your home and in yourself.

THROW OUT THE DEAD

Remove dried flower arrangements from your home immediately. All they are is *dead energy.* There is no life, only a stagnant remembrance of what was, a magnet for dust, and an obstruction of fresh, clean energy. As soon as you remove them, I am certain you will feel lighter; physically, mentally, and emotionally. If possible, replace them with live flowers. I am often asked if artificial plants or artificial flowers will suffice. I strongly feel that ersatz representations do not hold the same beauty, vibrancy, and vitality that live flora holds. Natural is always better than artificial. If you are surrounding yourself with artificial representations of beauty, what is that saying about yourself? Many times I have discovered homes where fake foliage prevailed and so has a feeling of superficiality. Yes, it does take time and dedication to remember to care for plant life, but those nurturing acts are significant ways to honor a living

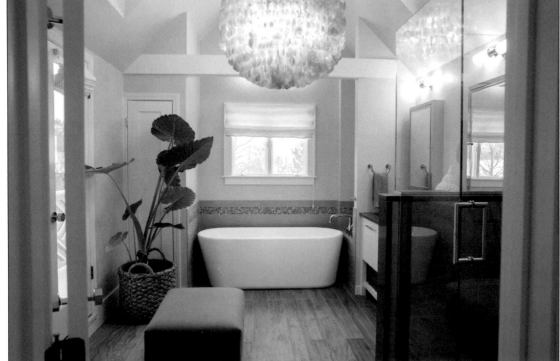

Courtesy of Olga Adler Interiors/ Debra Somerville Photography.

essence and to cultivate that karma within yourself and in your life. The energy feels much different in a home where tender loving care has been cultivated through attention to growth and development rather than just displaying the fruits of that labor in a fake representation that collects dust.

The Benefit of Plants

Plants are a great complement to any home and a suggestion I often make to clients. Some varieties filter indoor pollutants, and all increase the vitality and energy of a home. The Foliage for Clean Air Council recommends having "two plants for every 100 square feet." A two-year study with NASA scientists determined that "research has shown virtually every tropical indoor plant and many flowering plants are powerful removers of indoor air pollutants and several toxic chemicals from the air in building interiors. House plants also improve air quality by giving off water vapor and releasing oxygen." Make sure you add a thin layer of gravel on top of the dirt to cut down on possible mold.

Nearly every Feng Shui consultant would not recommend a cactus in a bedroom because of its "sha" chi (piercing arrows of chi, or energy, produced by sharp corners—in this case, the sharp needles). In each consultation, I've always believed that every situation needs individual consideration. In the separate bedrooms of a bedridden husband and healthy wife, this situation prevailed. The husband owned a twenty-year-old cactus that was a great source of strength for him. He felt that the cactus was a tough, hearty survivor—everything he was struggling to be. When he looked at that cactus, he felt physically powerful and resilient. I encouraged his wife to move the cactus into his room. It was previously just beyond the room and out of his line of sight from the bed. Having it closer made him feel more connected to the mighty energy he equated with its presence. A cactus symbolizes independence and strength. It perseveres in dry, unfavorable conditions. This is an example of how the psychological connections to symbols can be quite powerful and subjective. It's important that you check in with your own personal associations and only choose the objects that have the "right" meaning for you.

Plants are essential in your home, but if you feel you do not have a green thumb, ivy or snake plants are best because they have low water and light needs. I have heard all kinds of excuses from "I swear I will kill it," "I am so bad with plants," and "I don't have the time to water plants." In those cases, I suggest bamboo plants. All you have to do is stick them in enough water, avoid direct sunlight, and look at the water levels every couple months. Everyone can benefit from adding foliage in their home because these vibrant forces of life make an immediate difference in the ambient feel to a space. And anytime you can successfully bring splendors of nature inside to your living environment, it is beneficial for living. In addition, when toxic volatile organic compounds fill your home (dry-cleaning fluids, acetone, ammonia, detergents, plastics, paints, adhesives, etc.), your plants are not only scrubbing the air of these toxins, but they are doing something even a high-tech HVAC system

Pollutant	Sources	Solutions
Formaldehyde	Foam insulation, plywood, clothes, carpeting, furniture, paper goods, household cleaners	Philodendron Spider plant Golden pathos Bamboo palm Corn plant Chrysanthemum Mother-in-law's tongue
Benzene	Tobacco smoke, gasoline, synthetic fibers, plastics, inks, oils, detergents, rubber	English ivy Marginata Janet Craig Chrysanthemum Gerbera daisy Peace lily
Trichloroethylene	Dry cleaning, inks, paints, varnishes, lacquers, adhesives	Gerbera daisy Chrysanthemum Warneckei Peace lily Marginata

Source: Foliage for Clean Air Council, 405 N. Washington St., Falls Church, VA 22046.

can't: they are converting the volatile organic compounds (VOCS) into carbon-based materials in order to fuel photosynthesis. That means that the pretty peace lily and fluffy fern are actually reversing your carbon footprint while helping you breathe easier. And if that is not enough, the act of nurturing vibrant life sources in your home cultivates compassion in your environment.

The chart on page 76 shows the top ten plants in the NASA study that most effectively removed pollutants from the air.

YASMIN: CONTINUOUS CYCLES DISRUPTED

Yasmin rescheduled her consultation with me three times. First it was because of jet lag. Then it was because her new night shift work was throwing her off. Finally it was too much alcohol consumption on her birthday that made her oversleep. I found it worthy of note that all three reasons revolved around disruptions in her natural rhythmic cycles of sleep. When I finally did see her in the dead of winter, she seemed exhausted, depressed, and distracted. She wanted to focus on advancing her career, increasing her finances, improving her health, creating a general sense of balance, and saving for travel. First, I wanted to concentrate on getting her in sync with her natural, rhythmic Universal beat in order to get her on the fast track of clarity and the comfort and delight of synchronicity. Once that happens, then everything else can start to fall into place.

The more a person's biological cadence gets misaligned with the Tao, the more all kinds of conflict may occur. It's like constant Mercury in retrograde on high gear or a domino succession of unfortunate events. Whatever can go wrong, will. Your goals will seem further out of reach, and daily tribulations will bombard you with greater frequency. This can all set up a condition where eventually mental or physical ailments may occur. Yasmin's "out of sorts" challenges were throwing off not only her own inner clock, but her inner voice as well. Our bodies follow inherent biological clocks that we anticipate and adapt to. Sometimes it's the 24/7 clock. Or it's the okay-it's-dark-outside-it's-time-to-sleep clock. Sometimes we follow the pace of monthly cycles, seasonal cycles, cellular cycles, or more. Yasmin was not listening to her body and not giving herself what she needed most. She was skipping meals, eating junk food, not exercising, drinking alcohol in excess, and getting little sleep. All of these choices can take you further away from a pure channel to your higher self and get you off track from beautiful, shining moments of serendipity that guide you to your best potential.

Working nights as a nurse, Yasmin was having a hard time adjusting to the most counterintuitive cycle a human being can possibly endure—staying up nights and sleeping during the day. I kept my mind, body, and spirit suggestions mainly focused on optimizing the Universal cycles of nature in and around her. My first suggestion for her centered on creating an environment that would allow her to easily fall asleep during the day. This included a getting a sleeping mask and blackout drapes, moving her bed into a better position (more on positioning in chapter 5), and removing all active symbolism and extra electronics from her bedroom. In her living room and kitchen, I suggested lightbulbs that mimicked the natural waves of sunlight, so when she was up at night, she could assimilate more easily to being awake. Her apartment was lacking in fresh air. Even on cold days, I encouraged her to crack a window for circulation and get some air-cleaning plants or an air purifier. Sleep, sunshine, and fresh air—check, check, and check!

Next, I noticed that her surrounding elements throughout her home were as equally out of whack as she was. The Water and Fire elements were clashing side by side everywhere I looked: a water fountain on top of her fireplace, a jarring color scheme in her bedroom of red and black, and a black kitchen table that was triangular. These three examples all had Fire and Water in conflict. Wood is the buffer element between Water and Fire. (Water feeds Wood, Wood feeds Fire). The water fountain on her mantel was located in her Fame area. Since the Fame area connects to the element Fire, the water fountain was not in its power spot. Fire located in Fame will ignite your passion, enhance your reputation, and improve how you see yourself. Water was putting out all the Fire. A perfect location for it was in her entryway, which was the career area of her apartment. I recommended she paint and redecorate her bedroom in neutral tones and use green (the color that represents Wood) as an accent color. To balance it all out, doses of Metal and Earth were needed to complete the elemental flow in her home.

Yasmin was carrying the heavy energy of her sick patients home with her from the hospital where she worked. I told her about an old Feng Shui cure for releasing negative energy when leaving a hospital, cemetery, funeral parlor, or sick friend: do not go directly home. Stop somewhere first and visualize releasing any bad mojo you are holding on to before arriving home.

In the spring, I actually ran into Yasmin at a flea market. I barely recognized her. She looked glowing and vibrant. Even her mannerisms seemed lighter and more jubilant. She told me that her walks home through Central Park after work had become a therapeutic mind, body, spirit exercise that helped her the most. It was during this time that she would shed any depressing thoughts, go over a mental list of what she was grateful for, and look to "moments in nature" as a guide for the day. I asked her what exactly in nature would guide her. "Every day I would think about goals I wanted to accomplish and I would see something like a soaring oriole, a still turtle, bold squirrels . . . and I decided to take my daily cues on how to proceed from them. Recently, I'd kept noticing signs of new life. The bulbs shooting up through the dirt are kind of like me right now, on my way to a new beginning." Then Yasmin showed me her engagement ring and told me the details. I was glad she felt her life was coming together. Even though our consultation was not focused on finding a relationship, I knew that once she balanced the elemental deficiencies and excesses and aligned herself with the Universal forces around her, good things would begin to fall into place.

THE SPIRIT AND THE FIVE ELEMENTS

There are five spiritual expressions of the elements that are connected to your soul's purpose. The key to working with the Five Elements for spiritual growth is first to be able to clearly identify the root emotion that is the foundation for your current

Element	Related Emotion	Questions to Ask	Actions to Take
Water	Fear	What is the root of my fear? What do I need to feel trust?	Remove "I can't" or "I'm not" from your speech. Trust your choices, trust your decisions. Work on your intuition.
Wood	Anger	What is causing me to be so quick to anger? Why am I really feeling annoyed?	Know that every thought, feeling, and action carries a vibration. Tell yourself to take three long breaths when anger appears. Work on forgiveness and peace.
Fire	Joy	Am I lacking hope and love in my life? Do I feel a lack of gratitude?	Invite joy into your life by surrounding yourself with people who are positive and uplifting. Create reasons to celebrate. Work on living in the moment.
Earth	Sympathy	How do I help others who are in need? Is expressing compassion difficult for me?	Tell yourself that when you are apathetic to others, you are being that way to yourself. Recognize that others' experiences are connected to your own. Work on empathy and compassion.
Metal	Grief Sadness	Is my sadness caused by a particular event? Do I often feel alone?	Don't fight against thoughts of your loss or sorrow. Acknowledge them, then move forward by thinking of three things you are happy for. Know that you are not alone. Work on expressing yourself through movement or exercise.

spiritual lesson in this lifetime. Familiarize yourself with that elements' expression in your home and yourself.

When you worked on your clutter issues from the previous chapter, did any of the emotions from the table on pages 31–32 come up for you as to why you accumulate? If so, take your cues there. By now you most likely have discovered, for example, what element you are struggling with health-wise or what element you are avoiding using in your home. Whatever element keeps coming up for you, it's time to discover what the spiritual lesson is. If you are still not sure what emotion you may need to work on the most, ask yourself if a trusted loved one has ever pointed out that you have an excess, absence, or ongoing struggle with one of these emotions. Think about if you tend to draw in partners or friendships where this emotion is a dominating theme. The table below will help you.

In navigating your way through this process, as you reflect on the questions and implement the actions into your life, try to bring in some spiritual tools for help. With prayer, ask that whatever deity you connect to help you work with this emotion in order for you to transmute the negative lessons to a positive one. If meditation is your spiritual vehicle of choice, select one that focuses on that particular chakra. I like to work with my angels around me for guidance, to point me in the right direction for spiritual expansion by giving me a vital message for the day. Another way to spiritually connect and balance these Five Elements is to harness the energies of the actual element in nature. If you have the means, give it a try: sit under a tree to help adjust your Wood element, swim in the ocean for tweaking Water, hike on rock formations for Metal, plant your feet in the dirt for Earth, or sit near a fireplace for Fire.

Finding your groove means tuning in to your biological eternal rhythmic cycles, honoring the essence in all living things, and aligning yourself with nature to reach your maximum potential. The Five Elements can teach you how to strengthen and optimize your mind, body, spirit, and environment to help reach your goals, become healthier, live easier, and grow on a deeper level. By harnessing the literal and symbolic energies of these forces of nature, you can tap into their cycles to learn how to align yourself with a Universal flow. It is often when we are in sync with this energy that is within ourselves—yet greater than ourselves—when the Universe opens up with gifts to say, "Yes! You are on the right path!" For most people, when they are in sync with their Universal energy, there's a lot of happenstance that occurs. Coincidental events, dogged luck, fluke encounters all seem to act as beacons of encouragement that we are making good choices and we are right where we need to be. Sometimes, however, these turning points may reveal themselves as a seemingly negative situation. For me, my diagnosis felt like a destructive bomb that rocked my world. But not long after, I was yanked into this path where my mind, body, and spirit have flourished, I found my calling, and I have been able to help a few people along the way.

In the most important cycle of all, our lifetime, we go through many transformations in our own personal journey. Every component of our cycle—joy and grief, stillness and action, shortage and abundance, illness and health—gives us an opportunity for growth and evolution if we reflect on the wisdom that each teaches us. Sometimes this is not easy in the moment of a seemingly negative experience. How can you remember joy when a loved one has passed on? How can you feel secure when employment is lost and money is scarce? It is usually within these winter phases of stillness, scarcity, and darkness that you tend to learn and grow the most, especially if you are clear about your intentions, your goals, and your personal faith. Remember, always after winter comes the promise of new growth in the spring.

Now that you have cleared away the emotional, physical, and spiritual clutter, and you have your groove on, let's dig deeper and discover all the ways your subconscious issues are revealing themselves in your home.

CHAPTER FOUR

Go Deeper: Subconscious Symbolism in Your Home

"We have a hunger of the mind, which asks for knowledge of all around us, and the more we gain, the more is our desire; the more we see, the more we are capable of seeing."

—Maria Mitchell

Symbolism is constantly bombarding us. In religion, literature, movies, ceremonies, even traffic signage, we are continually receiving emblematic directions to guide and inform us in some way. Images in our home or office that we surround ourselves with can energetically weaken or strengthen our chi. Take a look at what images surround you in your home. Every object you see is energetically imbued with a meaning, whether you realize it or not. Collectibles, paintings, decorative objects, and photographs that we display all contain images that hold conscious and subconscious meanings for us. Ideally, we want to envelop ourselves with imagery that supports our goals and desires, allowing us to feel moved, inspired, comforted, or empowered.

Imagine if there was a device called a symbolism decoder that could examine aspects of your life that are dark, unclear, or problematic and draw direct correlations to your environment. Picture this device shifting the perceptions you hold regarding the connections between your environment and yourself. Once uncovered, these symbolic associations that mirror your personal story would enable you to live differently. *You are now that decoder.* By reading this book, you are already on your way to shifting your perspective on the meaning of your surroundings and realizing how their energy has a massive impact on your family, finances, health, opportunities, creativity, knowledge, reputation, career, and relationships.

Symbols and their meanings can differ culturally, socially, or psychoanalytically, but our responses to the symbolism of objects in our surroundings are individualized and depend heavily upon our experiences. At times, an object holds a universal meaning, and no extensive interpretation is necessary. For example, exercise equipment (like a treadmill or a stationary bike) conveys an image of fast movement and is not recommended for the bedroom. On a deeper level, it can also be a reminder of the exercise you did or didn't get to, and that can energetically prevent a peaceful night's rest either way. Pictures of crashing waves and sports cars do not belong in the bedroom either.

Sometimes the message can be up for interpretation depending on your experiences—a piece of furniture can have a different meaning for two people in the same household. One person sees the object as a comforting and familiar inherited object while the other sees it simply as an object to sit on, and that might be the extent of the significance. Most times, however, there are many items in our surroundings that can take on our energies, manifest our chi, and tell our stories on metaphysical levels.

EDITH: A MOUNTAIN OF INSPIRATION

Edith needed help setting up her home office. She was about to start a new home-based business. Among her artwork set aside for the room was a painting of Mount Kilimanjaro. I asked her what the painting meant to her. "The painting is called a Tinga Tinga. It is from Tanzania, and the reason Mount Kilimanjaro is so important to me is that it seemed like something completely impossible to do, but the impossible was achieved."

I wanted to know more and listened to her inspirational story.

"When my friend Cindy and I decided to go to Africa, it was not even a question— we were going to conquer Kili. Of course, we had no idea what we were getting into;

we didn't really even read up on it. We knew it was high, but not as arduous as colder climate climbs of the same altitude. All went fine for me until 18,500 feet. The altitude was getting to me, really slowing me down. It was one deep labored breath, followed by one step, leaning on my walking stick. I don't do anything slow in life . . . so this was a big challenge for me! I could see the peak—Uhuru—but given how I felt I became unsure I would make it. But then I reminded myself that I said I would get to the top. Cindy said to me, 'Just put one foot in front of the other.' At that moment I made the decision to overcome all of the physical sensations, exhaustion, and mental strain and focus on my breathing and move forward one step at a time. I got to the top only because I said I would. The painting means to me an adventurous exploration, being tenacious toward my goals, and doing exactly what I say I am going to do—no matter what."

The natural Feng Shui position for a mountain is behind you. I suggested she move her desk so that her back was to the painting. Placing a mountain image in *front* of you creates the feeling that life is a struggle and completion of tasks will require much effort. Facing that image will subconsciously imprint a degree of mental exertion throughout all your daily efforts, large or small. Landform Feng Shui practiced in ancient China states that a mountain at your back offers protection from the north winds and safety from enemy attacks. In this case, not only does the mountain image offer a feeling of protection, but also surmountable success, boosting a sense of achievement, making it the perfect reminder in a place for accomplishing new projects. Now, when Edith feels unsure about meeting a goal, she has the energetic resonance from that circumstance—consciously and subconsciously—right behind her, giving her the boost of confidence that she needs.

TONY AND JUDY: ELEVATING THE CHI, ELEVATING THEMSELVES

Tony and Judy had a deli and catering business for twenty years that was now in the red. No matter what they were doing, they could not seem to get ahead. A couple years after attending two of my lectures, they called me for a consultation for both their business and home. Utilities were shut off and put back on at a premium, back taxes were due, and contractors were owed. We sat in the tiny, closet-sized back office they divided with their bookkeeper and they shared the depths to which their finances and despair plummeted. "Our dreams are turning into a financial and emotional nightmare," Judy shared. Upon evaluating the business, the most significant reoccurring adjustment was to raise the base line of chi in every possible way throughout their business.

The symbolic literalism included changing out display shelves of packaged junk food for healthier choices that were better quality. "I was thinking about going with an organic snack vendor," Judy agreed. Processed food holds a lower vibration than healthier options. A more vibrant wall color was recommended to really make the menu boards pop, fluttering flags to catch attention from the road, and a higher wattage of lighting was necessary. Plants or flower sources were needed outside the door as you entered. In the future, if they could afford it, a superior quality countertop where patrons spent most of their time retrieving their coffee was recommended. Since the deli portion constituted only 30 percent of their sales, focus was made to raise the awareness and enhance the profile of the catering end.

I spotted a large sign that had the name of their catering business lying on the floor in the back room and recommended it be hung on the front of the catering desk where they took orders. It fit perfectly and seemed to herald this portion of the business loudly. It was important that this area be tended to with a new focus.

I created a new organizational system for taking and fulfilling orders by asking them to break down the steps of what happens when a new catering customer calls. Sometimes examining each step of a seemingly banal task and then questioning what's needed to efficiently complete it is the best way to create a new plan. In this case, a new system of hanging clipboards, a dry-erase board, and color-coded folder files were recommended. This area was the epicenter of the floor plan and the business. It needed to improve with artwork and design details. Both Tony and Judy were open to suggestions, took six pages of notes, and eagerly began to make adjustments in both locations right after the consultation. Right afterward, things got immediately worse for a short period of time. This is expected when powerful changes are newly made and the energy is shifted in any space. Energies get "shaken up" as the new adjustments take hold, and soon a steady and positive change usually begins to unfold.

With each month, their business began to increase and then reach record highs. Tony and Judy shifted their perspective when challenges came their way. They now faced challenges holistically, by connecting the psychological with the physical and the spiritual in creative ways. Fourteen months later, they asked me to come back to help them get to "the next level." They informed me that the apartment above their business was soon to be vacant, and as owners of this two-story building, they were concerned with getting a trustworthy tenant. When the suggestion was made to literally "take their office to a higher level" and move it out of the overcrowded closet downstairs to a larger space above the business, the symbolism resonated well with them and just felt right. They immediately had ideas of asking other associates in the catering business—DJs, photographers, wedding planners—to rent a room in the space, which could lead to a bountiful network of referrals within the group.

"From now on, when you enter this lot every day, think of it as your catering *headquarters*! Your business has expanded, and so must your office. Now you will have physically and symbolically moved to a higher level!" I told them. An important factor here was creating the space for expansion, which allows the growth to happen more easily. Setting the intention for growth reinforces the physical with the mental. Months later, they informed me that instead of renting out the remaining upstairs office space to their industry peers, they chose to let a couple of their employees live there who were going through a difficult time. To me, this heartfelt choice held a more meaningful, energetic repercussion that would continue to enhance their chi and good fortune as time went on.

SAMMY: COMPLETELY SURROUNDED AND ALL ALONE

In a client's biography I received before the consultation, the words "in a room full of people, I often feel alone" kept coming back to me while I studied the floor plan. It wasn't until I was inside the home did I realize why he would feel that way. Every single room displayed dozens and dozens of framed photographs of people—from famous faces to distant acquaintances and loved ones. Standing in the kitchen, I felt the sense of loneliness around me. There must have been a hundred eyes looking at me. Too many to feel intimate; it felt more like a group that I was not a part of. Hallways were salon-style with more photographs, leading to more rooms with the same amount of pictures. Once the obvious correlation between his dilemma and his surroundings was pointed out, he paused and was momentarily silent. Then I saw a spark of recognition in his eyes. He quickly began removing some pictures.

At a follow-up consultation a year later, his home looked completely different, and loneliness was not an issue. The opposite was occurring. Sammy's love life was busy, but he wondered why he could not have a committed relationship. He said he wanted nothing more than to fall in love with someone special. In our walk-through of his space, women's perfume was heavy, female toiletries were all over the bathroom, and high heels were strewn about in his closet. He acknowledged that they were from "various women I'm dating."

"Sammy, how do you think a potential girlfriend would feel coming into your home and seeing reminders like this everywhere?" I asked as I pointed to the women's panties hanging from the stationary bike. He laughed but gathered some of the items up and agreed. I explained the importance of adjusting your environment to be in complete alignment with your goals. I silently wondered if Sammy really wanted a committed relationship or just thought it would be the "right" thing to profess. Either way, I encouraged him to spend some solo time working on his internal environment (his thoughts and goals) and his spatial one (his home) so they could mirror one another more truthfully. It's quite common, when you are living in it, not to see the direct connections. Sammy's issues happened to be blatant signs that emerged easily on the surface. Sometimes, the signs are hidden and not so transparent.

HIDDEN SYMBOLISM

Many times, our deeper "stories" are not necessarily found in objects that are purposely displayed. Closets can represent our hidden emotional problems. Similar to the recesses of our mind, these concealed chambers mirror our obscured issues that we choose to not deal with. Like when the company is about to arrive and there is a last-minute toss of miscellaneous items into these welcoming collection pits. We are hiding what we don't want others to see. When closets or drawers are permanently jam-packed messes and the house is otherwise tidy, the underlying emotional issues tend to be more deeply hidden. Insecurity and fear play a big role in the secret-semi-hoarder's life. (See chapter 7 for more on how fear shows up in your home.)

A client kept telling me she "could not get a handle on things no matter what she did." She felt overwhelmed and anxious most of the time. As I stood in her kitchen and looked around, there were no knobs on any of her drawers! She said she took off the old knobs after she purchased new ones, but the new ones didn't fit, and she didn't want to put the old ones back on. So for over one year, she struggled daily to get into her cabinets and drawers. The constant awkwardness of uneasily grasping exacerbated her feeling of "not being able to get a handle on things" in other areas of her life. Years later, while relating this exact story to a client with similar life challenges to explain how symbolism manifests in a space, she told me, "That is precisely what I have going on with my drawers!" The more consultations I have done, the more I have witnessed that these examples are quite common and usually every household has at least one. Yes, that means you.

Examine Symbolism in Your Own Home

When a visible manifestation in imagery occurs like this, it is helpful to examine the process of how it began. Did your current *life circumstance* (in the case above, not getting a "handle" on life) subconsciously dictate the physical representation in the surroundings? Or, did the *imbalanced surroundings* (no handles) come first and are the source of that growing emotional issue? Essentially, you are the conduit of expression for your living space. Either an existing symbolic issue in your home will eventually mirror that matter in your life or your problems in life will start to symbolically show up in your living space. By examining how the channel of imbalance appears, either expression in your home can reveal more about your life, your responsiveness to your home surroundings, and how well you manage challenges.

I have helped many clients who are greatly in tune or sensitive to their environment. If you already know you are this way, it's another reason to tackle domestic disruptions like home repairs and disorganization quickly. If there are reoccurring patterns of negative emotions in your life, try to look for parallels of how that emotion is characteristically showing up in your space.

MY STORY: HOLISTICALLY READING SYMBOLISM

The moment my consultation ended on a new Fifth Avenue four-bedroom apartment, my client, Viviane, exclaimed, "My husband and our architect will be relieved to hear that you did not recommend any brass wind chimes, Foo dogs, or red walls! You are the first Feng Shui consultant to come in here and not do that. Why?"

I explained to her that only after my extensive Feng Shui training, and hundreds of clients spanning over a decade, have I realized how to effectively utilize and translate the same principles of influencing the chi in ways that my clients can relate to. Viviane's apartment was very modern with white walls and clean lines. Even all the electrical switch plates were flush-mounted so as to not interrupt the extreme seamless look, which was paramount in the architectural details and style of the home.

Their sleek and clean preferences were evident everywhere. A red wall in the middle of their creamy monochromatic showplace would stick out like a sore thumb and disconnect continuity for their entire home. Firecrackers, dragons, and Foo dogs would disrupt their design concept even further and make them feel annoyed every day to look at them. Those culturally rich items were not symbols that they related to. Part of my job is to read the energy of my clients along with their spaces and make recommendations in alignment with both. As this chapter teaches, the dominating factor is *your own personal authentic association* to these objects, colors, and symbols.

If you need to activate the chi inside your home, perhaps a traditional consultant would recommend hanging wind chimes in several places (like Viviane's previous consultant suggested), but in this case I recommended vibrant life forces of hearty plants and orchids. Another symbolic adjustment included slowing down the chi in one long hallway, for which I recommended a patterned rug and framed pictures on the wall. One of Viviane's priorities was to feel more secure and less scattered. I suggested that some overly fragile glass tables could be swapped out for more solid ones, and area rugs were desperately needed to ground the space in the living room and bedroom. As with all recommendations, I connect the mind, body, and spirit into my client's space for the greatest transformations. For example, it's not just adding a plant to your space and calling it a day. It's connecting to how plants are vibrant visual reminders of beauty and life (mind). It is knowing that they are working hard at removing indoor pollutants and are helpful to your health (body). By engaging in their cultivation, plants nurture compassion within your environment and yourself (spirit).

To help increase their wealth in the wealth gua, I went with encouraging them to purchase investment pieces that were strong and solid and reminders of their own stable prosperity—not a frog statue with a coin in its mouth. They could not even bear to make that purchase, which an earlier Feng Shui expert recommended. In the same way that you would not want an overly persuasive interior designer dictating how your home will look, you don't want a Feng Shui consultant doing the same. A good Feng Shui consultant will offer multiple options that in the end have the same result of tweaking the energy where needed, but complementing your aesthetic. I take it further, with the mind, body, spirit, space connections that personalize these energetic suggestions and lead to a deeper transformation, and now you can, too.

Symbolism is one mighty force. It can affect you more than you are aware of. It's important to carefully examine not just the energy of the items that surround you, but also the symbolic energy of your actions in your home, too. Do you really need to watch the late-night news before you go to bed and bombard your brain with mostly horrific imagery and negative information? When you get up in the morning, are you setting the tone for a prepared day by making your bed? Are you making time to sit down and eat dinner with your family regularly? Are you honoring your space by taking time to keep it somewhat clean when you can? Allow your routines in your home to carry these symbolic concepts through a whole-system approach that combines your thinking, your body, your feelings, and your space, all together. Doing so will always be more effective in the end.

HOLISTICALLY TACKLING SYMBOLISM— THE MIND, BODY, SPIRIT, SPACE WAY

If you look around your own home and don't see how your life challenges are symbolically manifesting around you, think of the words or phrases that you use regularly to describe them. Feel like you are always "up against a wall"? Check to see if your bed is literally up against a wall on one side or if, upon entering your home, you quickly face a wall. If so, move the bed so you have walking space on both sides. If space is tight, at the very least have a bit of breathing room on the wall side. If you face a wall within a few steps upon entering your front door, add a mirror to that wall.

In many consultations, I commonly hear a "life is passing me by" theme. If you feel you don't have the time to either pay the bills or follow your bliss, take a close look at your levels of organization. Simply not dwelling efficiently in your space can take up a chunk of your time. If you are constantly looking for your keys, taking longer to get dressed, or dreading going through the big pile of bills that has amassed, you are wasting valuable time that could be spent otherwise.

"Not having enough energy" is another one. When I hear that, I immediately look at the energy of the home. Clutter and tchotchkes can impede the flow of chi. A bed on the floor can suck your own life force. Lift it up with risers or even wood blocks so you have a clear path of chi under your bed. Low lighting throughout your home can mean low energy. Increase all lightbulb wattage, and keep lights on longer. Studies have shown that the scent of lemons or grapefruit is uplifting. Take an aromatherapy lemon bath, or just keep a bowl of lemons on display regularly and add a slice to your water. Does your home feel alive? A lively home is bursting with chi from plants, flowers, a water feature, music, candles, or pets. An alive home is as organic as possible with filtered air that circulates freely and has little to no off-gassing from heavy plastic and vinyl loads. An alive home is not a hub for over-consumerism that taxes the planet. The quickest way to make your home feel alive is to make sure you have air circulating. If you can't crack a window, at least keep a ceiling fan on low. Open the drapes or blinds during the day to let sunshine filter in; even if you are gone all day and you feel it doesn't matter, it does!

Feel like you can't "see an important issue clearly"? Check to see if your windows—which represent the eyes in Feng Shui—are clear. Make sure that your windows and all surfaces are sparkling clean. One client was having trouble making a pivotal career decision. Upon examining her career gua, I saw that there was a window inside her overflowing coat closet (put there to give a symmetrical look to the front exterior of the house). The window in the closet was sealed permanently shut and covered with a dingy curtain. Facing the curtain was a rack of coats. I recommended that she clean and unseal the window (yet always have it locked for safety), remove the curtain, and re-situate the coats so that they did not completely cover the window. It is essential when you are making these adjustments to set your intention and envision the change you hope to see in your life. While moving the bed, visualize that you now have more successful options in life. While adding the mirror, focus on the limitless, positive possibilities that are there for you. In cleaning any reflective surface in your home, reflect on issues that you need clarity on. And finally, examine your speech. Instead of saying "I never have enough time," change that to "I have plenty of time." No more "I don't have enough energy." Make it: "I have more than enough energy!" Our words are powerful.

Examining your symbolic challenges is the mind part; adjusting your surroundings is the action or the physical aspects that are the body. The spirit part is the visualizations of creating the outcome you desire and, in this case, realizing the energetic strength of the power of words.

SYMBOLISM IN RELATIONSHIPS

The most common and visible illustrations of imagery in homes that I see relates to relationships. Good or bad, imbalanced or well-adjusted, missing or present, the warnings, harbingers, or inequities in relationships can physically come to the forefront rather noticeably. A good percentage of the consultations that I go on revolve around concerns in this area. Everyone has them—from strengthening existing relationships to bringing in new ones to getting rid of old ones.

I witnessed a loved one go through a painful divorce and was shocked to hear that during this course of action, she was keeping the large framed wedding picture of her and her soon-to-be ex under her bed. At best, there should be nothing under the bed, but if space is a necessity, neat storage boxes with neutral objects like bedding or clothing are acceptable. The bed represents marriage and relationships. Whatever you have underneath it will energetically be vibrating that much closer to you when you are sleeping and at your most vulnerable state. The impact will be much more profound. When I pointed out the significance of this, these were her responses:

"The frame is beautiful and I love it."

"But it is wrapped up in Bubble Wrap."

"I plan on using that same frame for a picture of me and my new boyfriend."

It is not uncommon for defenses and excuses to come in to play when symbolism is pointed out like this. Intending to exchange the "framework" from a failed relationship to a brand-new one can be detrimental for the new relationship. It does not matter if the picture is wrapped in Bubble Wrap or in a lead box under the bed. The symbolic presence of such an emotionally charged image is very powerful. Keeping items from previous relationships—especially under the bed—hinders all the best to unfold in current relationships. Unhealthy patterns can have a propensity to be repeated or developed, and growth can be stagnated. In this case, jumping from one relationship to another *within the same framework* literally mirrored the inability to break relationship patterns or examine oneself. Nothing I shared about the energetic ramifications of having a large picture of an ex under your bed—*especially when you are trying to establish another relationship*—resonated with her. And that's okay. Ralph Waldo Emerson was often attributed as saying, "People only see what they are prepared to see."

Understandably, not everyone will be open to having their darkest secrets or unhealthy patterns revealed and pointed out to them. It can feel like a spotlight is shining on your weaknesses, and it can be painful and difficult to accept. In time, hopefully the imagery will make its way out of the house (as it did here), but if you are not ready to do the work on yourself, the connections will seem insignificant. Examining your surrounding symbolism will seem like nonsense, and the ego and immediate consciousness will do everything to discount and dismiss this information. Circumstances might even become unpleasant if you see something like this and try to point it out to the person you are intending to help if they did not *ask* for this information. From that moment on, I have not given unsolicited Holistic Home advice. Make sure you don't either. (Just give this book, instead!)

MARCY: LIFE AFTER GRIEF

Letting go is never easy. In one consultation, my heart was full of empathy for Marcy's heartbreak. A year and a half earlier, she found her husband of thirty-five years dead in their bathroom from a heart attack. She was cautiously trying to start dating but felt guilty in pursuing it. I immediately urged her to get rid of the king-size mattress she had shared with her husband and purchase a new queen- or full-size one. Whenever there is sickness, change of partners, or death it is wise to start fresh with a new mattress as soon as possible.

I mentally superimposed the bagua map in her living room. In her relationship area was a dead Christmas tree from *the year before* when her husband passed away. She knew it should go but she was having a very difficult time removing it. This was the last object her husband touched before he died. He was in the midst of taking it down by clipping the branches off from the bottom up and all that remained was a few upper layers. He had joked about how funny it looked at that point and left it that way on purpose. Depending on the moment when relaying this story, Marcy could either laugh or cry. As much as I saw this tree as an energetic emotional anchor for her, I was not about to instruct her to remove it right then. She knew it had to go, but it had to be when *she* was ready. After we did a clearing and blessing ceremony in her home, I explained the importance of what the tree symbolized in her healing and grieving process and that once she removed it, it would be a lot easier for her to move forward in the areas she needed.

Executing change is the biggest block that most clients encounter during and after a consultation. Change represents the unknown. Stepping out of your comfort zone and delving into areas where you do not feel secure and at ease is not an action that most would seek out and embrace. It certainly takes a brave leap of faith to trust that these recommended holistic changes could ultimately serve you well—even if sometimes that change initially causes discomfort, fear, or stress.

BARBARA AND RICARDO: A RELATIONSHIP MADE FOR ONE

Barbara had been dating Ricardo for over a year and was unhappy with how the levels of commitment were progressing. She was ready for a deeper sense of devotion from him and when the topic came up, he seemed despondent and not ready to make the commitment she desired. Walking through her bedroom, this is what I saw: Her headboard and bedside were both pushed up against walls. A pillow on her bed had an embroidered image of a single woman. One single chair sat in the far right corner. Her closet was packed with her clothes and accessories with no room to spare. Solitary items such as a singular vase, a lone figurine, and a single glass heart were dispersed throughout her room. Artwork and photographs were all single images. One nightstand sat on her side of the bed.

The bedroom is the energetic abode for relationships. It did not surprise me that her boyfriend lacked the desire to commit. From just examining the physical symbolism, there simply was no room for him. Only place the headboard to the wall. Avoid pushing one of the sides of your bed up against the wall. The person who is sleeping on that side will feel claustrophobic—literally up against the wall with nowhere to go. There should be an open flow of chi all around the bed. The single imagery all generated an environment densely created for one. In the *relationship* corner of her bedroom sat one lone chair. Besides Ricardo feeling that there was subconsciously no place for him in this relationship, perhaps Barbara was truly not ready for creating a permanent space for Ricardo!

When intending to focus on a relationship, items should be paired in twos while visualizing the relationship evolving in the direction you desire. The closet had no room for Ricardo. If he were to stay over, there was no space for him to even hang a shirt. Make space for your partner—even if you don't have a relationship yet but want one in your life! Create room in the closet, a drawer in the bureau, a section in the medicine cabinet, and even space in the refrigerator. Once the space is literally and metaphorically made available, improvements will occur. Not only are you making space for your partner, but for your own growth as well. In order to bring a functional and healthy relationship into your life, it takes work on an emotional, spiritual, and physical level.

By addressing the physical issues of your space and the representation of your chosen items, it leads you to address the emotional and spiritual matters behind them. Some people may be ready to move the bed but not their point of view. Once Barbara dealt with the superficial, physical adjustments, she was forced to deal with the weightier issues that came to the surface right after, yet she had trouble doing so. Barbara emailed me, "Relationship issues are more prominent now. It's like I can't hide from them. I feel like I'm forced to deal with his issues and . . . I don't want to." They got engaged shortly after then called it quits for good. Barbara got in touch years later when she emailed me with a question but still seemed to lack the self-awareness of her own role in the demise of the relationship, as she still extensively blamed Ricardo for everything that went wrong. Making holistic adjustments helped bring Barbara to the point of addressing the issue, but if you don't want to continue the process, the issues won't just go away. They will lurk under the surface and continually impede healthy progress going forward.

KATHLEEN: ON THE SURFACE IT'S GREAT; SUBCONSCIOUSLY, NOT SO MUCH

With surprising frequency, I have worked with numerous clients who do not create enough room for their partners. Kathleen, a cosmetics executive who recently bought her own apartment, gushed in her bio about her and her boyfriend's incredible relationship and how in love they were. He was supposed to be moving in with her, but he was not available for the consultation. Once inside her space, there was no trace of him and no room in the closet for any of his things. She told me he was

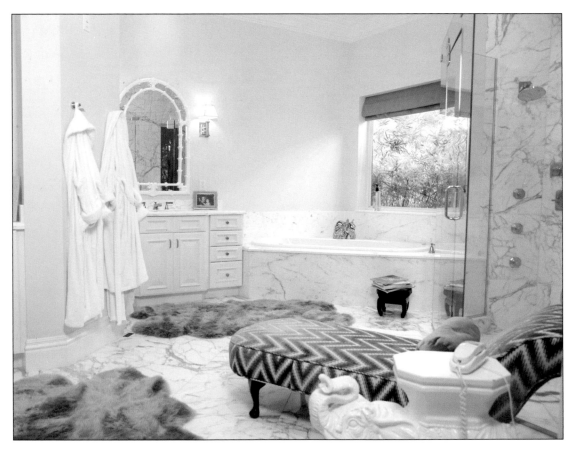

A private master bathroom shared by a couple is a perfect place to enforce twosome energy with their photograph and side-by-side robes.

spending less and less time with her and more time at his home upstate. She added that he was hesitant to bring in his belongings because he worked so much. I asked, "Where can he hang up his suits? Does he even have a drawer? Anything?" She said there was some hanging space in the hall closet. I looked. It was about three inches wide. Even though she was saying the relationship was great, her subconscious was shouting an even louder message: I'm not ready for this. (Or possibly: He's not ready for this and I know it.)

I gave many action-oriented recommendations that centered on making him a stronger presence in the apartment. It would require him to step up and proactively claim some space. One task involved going furniture shopping together and getting his input on all the remaining pieces they still needed. I told her that a lukewarm "Whatever you like, honey, is fine" would not be a sufficient response. He needed to actively try creating a space in both the relationship and the apartment. If this mission were followed, this course of action would then compel primary relationship issues to the forefront.

I don't know if the tasks and recommendations were implemented, but I do know that a couple months later they broke up. Two years later she sold the apartment, got married to someone else, and moved to Los Angeles. She recently emailed me asking for nursery room tips.

CHELSEA: AN UNREMARKABLE "ONE NIGHT STAND" RELATIONSHIP

On a consultation with Chelsea, I noticed her nightstand: a rather large side table, artfully arranged with flowers, lighting, and a couple books. Nightstands symbolically represent the equality in a relationship. They should be symmetrical and equivalent in size and shape. When one is missing, dominant, or inferior to the other, the relationship has the potential to mirror that imbalance as well. An overpowering nightstand usually belongs to the dominant one in the relationship and a smaller

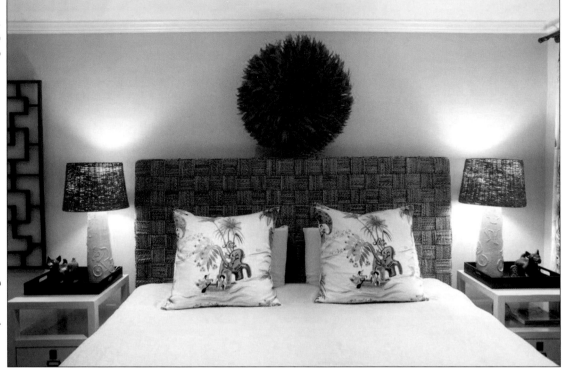

Courtesy of Olga Adler Interiors/Debra Somerville Photography

Ideally, nightstands should be somewhat equal in size, content, and quality, being that they symbolically represent an equal balance in partnerships. Here, the addition of an image of a couple in the tropics on the pillows enhances a playful pairing.

one to the submissive one. The nightstands can be different in style, but should be relatively matched in size and quality.

Chelsea's new boyfriend's side of the bed had the teeniest, round table I had ever seen, which held a very small table lamp with no bulb. His nightstand was bare and wobbly. The headboard was unstable and not secured behind the bed. Her bio, which I received before the consultation, did not indicate any problems in her relationship. "Tell me about the current situation between you and your boyfriend."

"He is out of the country right now and we are contemplating our future. He is much younger and we have issues about him not feeling financially equal in our relationship."

Intuitively I felt that the relationship had already ended, but did not want to share that. Instead I pointed out the significant disproportion in the nightstands and the shaky headboard and how that represents relationship balance and stability. She was not aware that she had arranged the furniture to parallel their current state and was concerned about him feeling inadequate *because* of this set up. "Why did I do this? Do I subconsciously see him as inferior?" Chelsea sat on the bed and reflected on the rickety setup that was heavier on the shabby than the chic. "This is an unremarkable one-night stand," she glumly concluded. (Or, *one* unremarkable *nightstand*, I smiled to myself.) Did she unknowingly create this atmosphere because that dynamic was already imbued in the matrix of their relationship? Or, did she just happen to not put any thought into his side of the bed? Both scenarios could have elements of truth and are worth exploring. One thing is certain, however: once symbolism is pointed out and brought to the forefront, it is very difficult to keep things the same if you truly want a change in your life. She knew the relationship was going through shifts, and once she made the energetic adjustments in her bedroom for a more balanced outcome, it quickly brought their relationship to an end when he returned. The relationship could not vibrate in tandem with the new energetic fine-tuning.

Once recommended adjustments are put into action, and intentions are applied, energics will adjust to support the desired outcome for the higher good. Sometimes these changes may not be what you think you want or need at the time. But in the long run, it almost always works out for the better. I was happy and a little surprised to hear that only two weeks later another man came into her life. Chelsea reported that he was just like her new nightstands—an equal match.

I cannot stress the importance of this connection enough. I have not come across this association much in my Feng Shui studies—however, time and time again, I have personally seen this illuminating, symbolic illustration of relationship inequality existing in homes dealing with the same. If this is what's lurking in your bedroom, you know what to do. Transparent, symbolic examples like this one are quite common, and usually every household has at least one. What is yours?

HEATHER AND MAX: THE APARTMENT THAT TEACHES

When Heather and Max contacted me for a consultation in the spring of 2003, they lived in a one-bedroom apartment and had recently had a baby. Their newborn was having some problems. Her eye was constantly running and clogged with mucus, and she was also having trouble sleeping. They often tried to rearrange things in search of harmony but nothing felt right. Necessary repairs always seemed to center around the flooring and foundation of their home. Relationships with their families and finances were strained. They gave up their bedroom for the baby and moved their own bed into the dining room, using a screen divider to create a makeshift master bedroom. Their sex life had slowed down, and Heather had low energy. Their main goal was to someday buy a two-bedroom apartment.

There were a few symbolic adjustments that needed to be made immediately. Babies' rooms are important places to apply holistic adjustments because children are so impressionable to the energies of their spaces. Energetic imbalances will be much more amplified to the growing, sensitive spirits of children. In Feng Shui, the windows represent the eyes and the ability to see things clearly. In their daughter's room, there was one window that remained unclean, with thick, visible layers of dirt and grime. When I inquired as to why only that one window was dirty when the others in the apartment were not, they replied that that window was inaccessible whereas all other windows could be reached and cleaned easily from a terrace. In this case, the dirty window had a direct energetic connection to her eye ailment and needed to be tended to. Their building had a window cleaning service that could access that window immediately. Rushing chi—such as the direct pathway into the baby's room—should not be met with a crib. The crib had to be moved to a more protected position that was not in direct alignment of the doorway, yet could be seen upon entering the room.

Heather and Max's improvised bedroom lacked a sense of stability and security. They did not have a door or a headboard. Headboards symbolize the stability of a marriage and should always be strong, sturdy, and securely fastened. The doorless bedroom enhances a sense of impermanence and vulnerability. In addressing Heather's low energy, lighting was increased throughout the home, because darkness can lead to depression and lethargy. I recommended that they hang brass chimes over the front door to activate the energies of the house and to play stimulating music often. Any mirrors that cut off views of the head can cause headaches, so they were adjusted to reflect a whole image. Heather often used aromatherapy, so I recommended lemon to refresh and uplift.

The wealth area of their home lacked abundance. This section was empty and dark. Plants were suggested as well as incandescent lighting pointing upward. This position for lighting directs the flow of chi in an uplifting way. Plants are a powerful life force that add vitality and can enliven any living space. Extra light was suggested to illuminate the wealth areas both literally and metaphorically. Whatever areas of your life need clarity or focus, find the correlating gua and add additional light. Literally shine light on it. However, be mindful that whatever area you are illuminating, dark issues might be first to come to light. If lighting already exists there, increase the wattage, and leave the lights on longer than you usually might. Increased lighting raises the chi.

Repairs on the foundation of their apartment were as endless as the maintenance on the actual foundation of their lives—their family history. Both constantly struggled with family issues and dynamics ingrained from a lifetime of dysfunctional behavior put upon them. If they were reaching an emotional breakthrough with a family member, or enduring another family-related obstacle, symbiotically their foundation problems would ebb and flow with the same vibration.

Through the following years, as they made changes, they made the mind, body, spirit connections in their space. They applied intention and used visualizations of their family ties, careers, and finances being strengthened. They developed a deep connection with their environment and began to clearly see on their own the connections between their space and their symbolic associations to themselves. Soon, the family was expanding again with another baby, and at the same time a bigger space they hoped for became available in their building. It needed some work but was within their budget. Heather and Max felt the holistic adjustments they did together brought them to the new space they were now ready for. "We did all we could in that space. We grew in many ways and are now ready to expand," they told me.

Heather and Max now had a heightened sense of awareness of their own environment. They were already making renovations with intention, choosing colors and décor with purpose, and meaningfully placing their objects and furniture.

Then one day I received an email from Heather detailing her frustration with the new apartment. The new wood floor was improperly installed, new appliances were damaged, orders were incomplete, incorrect supplies were delivered, and problems with the co-op board began to develop. She felt that she and Max had to unfairly take responsibility for all the improper structural work done by the former tenants, which led to a leak in their bathroom and was now causing damage to the apartment below. After that, a vent cover shot out of the wall and hurt Max's leg. A plumbing leak can represent two things in Feng Shui: finances or emotional issues. The former tenants of their new apartment really symbolized their parents. The substandard plumbing work represented the shoddy emotional work that had been done to them. Heather and Max were responsible for how it trickled down to the apartment below in the same way that they are now responsible for their own emotional issues trickling down to their offspring. Like the shooting vent cover, it has the potential to cause damage if not dealt with in an effective manner.

After endless structural work, they had to settle for a slightly uneven floor. In starting a family, your own childhood becomes that much more relevant in knowing what you do and don't want to do as a parent. "Our families did not give us a good foundation and we don't have anything to go back on, to draw from," Heather said. They were both working so hard to not pass down the dysfunction they grew up with to their children. This issue was constantly on the forefront of their consciousness, therefore on the forefront of their surroundings as well.

I encouraged them to see their apartment as their loving teacher. It came to them when they were expanding their family as well as their own consciousness, and issues were being forcibly transported to the surface. The apartment became the driving force behind their need for personal change, taking the hits, assisting them in their journey, and teaching them along the way with a blatant richness in symbolism. I advised them to change their perspective. Go from victim to empowered recipient. "Once you revel in the valuable lessons here, you will feel liberated and wiser. Gratitude is the message. Thank your space for the lessons you are receiving just as you would other gifts in your life. Even if the lessons are painful, that's when the most growth can occur." Five years later, Heather and Max sold their place and have been renting a house with a yard that their—happily adjusted—kids are enjoying.

CASE STUDY: SUSAN FASANO

Co-owner of Hamptons West, a chic boutique of cool home goods in West Sayville, New York, Susan Fasano says this dining table vignette in her home (featured on

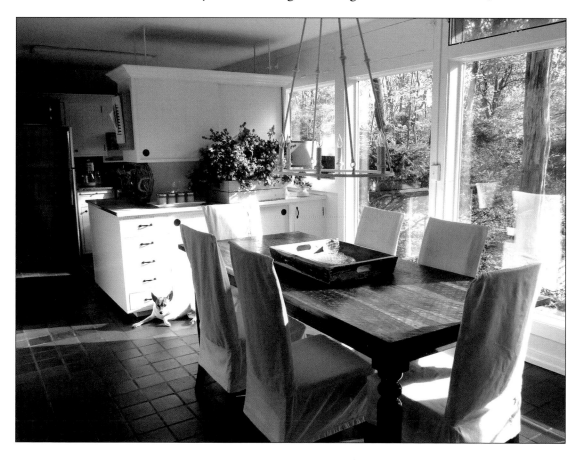

pages 105–107) symbolizes her perfectly. "My farm table was a great find that I gaily dragged back from Florida. I love my tray so much because my brother, who is a trained chef, taught himself carpentry and made it from reclaimed wood. My chair covers are made from old curtain panels. The Depression-era glass is a collection that my mother gave me before she passed away. And the light fixture was a quick DIY piece from Home Depot that I painted white and removed the shades. A transformation and collection of simple things that make me happy!

"Although my initial interest in weathered items and distressed furniture began with, 'Look at what nature has produced,' that led to a curiosity of its provenance. Where did it come from? Who may have handled it? Or, look at what someone has put curbside for me to rescue and give new life," says Fasano.

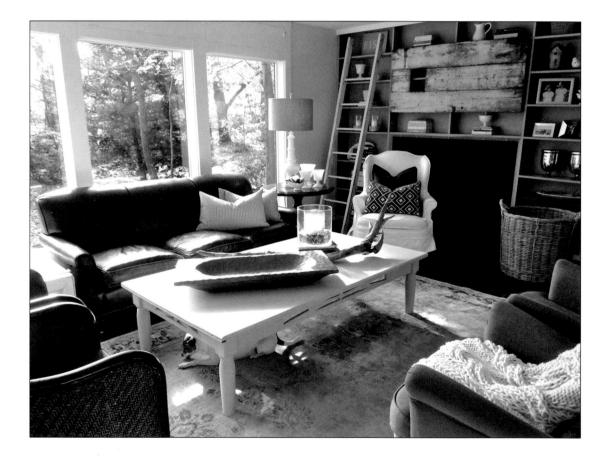

"Now, combining that concept with the sheer practicality of living in a stylish and comfortable home with children and pets came the birth of my rustic home with items that certainly carry a lot of personal significance to me. I learned a long time ago that things will never be perfect. Life is not perfect. So the challenge was how to make it inviting, affordable, and charming at the same time." Susan could not find a coffee table large enough, so she cut the legs off of a dining table and painted it white.

All types of relationship issues—from self, to partner, to family—tend to manifest in symbolic ways in our homes. Symbolism illustrates how each person can project characteristics onto objects or patterns in the home that represent their challenges in both conscious and subconscious ways. Examination of personal interpretation

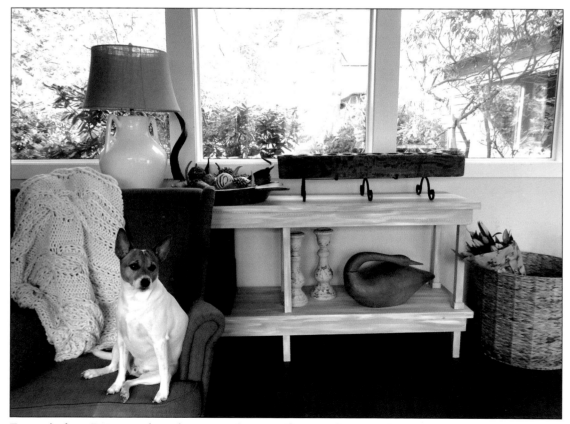

Fasano's dog, Raj, somehow becomes the star of every photograph.

can bring a deeper understanding of your inner emotional life, drawing awareness to specific areas that might require growth and shifts in perspectives. It is only when we look below the surface that we can begin to experience life more fully. Now, let's discover how you can position yourself for the best to develop in your life.

CHAPTER FIVE

Get in Position! Rule the World from Where You Sit, Stand, and Sleep

"Action is the foundational key to all success."

—Pablo Picasso

Tina and Mitch were together for six years and were engaged. Both were married before, and each had two children. Mitch recently moved into Tina's home where she had lived for the past twenty-four years, and during that time—while living in that same house—she was married and divorced twice. Mitch's children came to live with him and Tina every other weekend and more often during the summertime. One challenge was merging the two families in ways that the four children, as well as the stepparents, would feel comfortable. There were tension and arguments erupting among the children. There was one clear theme that kept coming up in this consultation: positioning. The physical importance of positioning throughout the home was as significant as what "position" each person would play in this new, uncertain dynamic of an extended family unit.

Walking through Tina and Mitch's home, I saw family divides in multiple longitudes throughout their home. The first one was the dining room table, where some arguments between two stepsiblings had recently occurred. A rectangular table with seating for six regularly sat Mitch's two children on one side of the table and

Tina's two children on the other side. An invisible line could be drawn down the middle for his and her sides. I suggested they mix it up by blending the stepsiblings next to one another. I also recommended that recessed lighting above the table be removed and changed for one central light fixture that illuminated everyone evenly, not just singular spotlights on some.

The second floor had three bedrooms: the master bedroom and a bedroom for each of Tina's children. Mitch's children each had their own bedroom too—but it was down in the semifinished and dark basement. Even though Mitch's kids were only there part-time, I felt that the underground floors were enforcing the line of delineation between families. Structurally, options were limited. Moving Tina's kids or doubling up the kids and having two per room upstairs was not an option (doubling up had been tried unsuccessfully once before), so the bedrooms had to stay where they were.

Bedrooms located in basements can feel oppressive with their below-ground location, lower ceilings, and diminished natural light. Basements, or any living space where the chi is stifled like this, can benefit from an air purifier, more lighting, flowers, plants, or an aquarium to liven up the space and start the activation of good flowing chi. The family needed a central location to congregate where they could play games and watch television. My solution was to create a family room space in the basement between the two bedrooms, which would physically and metaphorically bring the family down to the area where the other two kids (who felt the most neglected in this setup) were located. This new meeting place brought the higher floor occupants closer to the ones on the lower level and created an energetic anchor for all. I also noted that there were no photographs of the entire family displayed in the house. They were aware of this but added it to their list of adjustments and intended to change it as soon as possible. Adding these pictures of the family would be a perfect complement to the dining area and the new family room.

Position. The word itself can have a range of meanings. A holistic perspective takes it one step further. Besides the direction or way an object is placed, it can mean one's opinion and attitude as well as one's ranking in a family, company, or group. What I have discovered is that each definition of this word can have a direct meaning and connection to literal arrangements of your physical position in your home or work environment. Mitch and Tina were dealing with the ramifications of a household adjusting to its new roles and shifts in the extended familial unit. Raising awareness of positions for key elements such as bedrooms and even dinner table seating arrangements was an essential step in setting up a supportive environment. Once it was clearly pointed out how the children's deeper emotional concerns of position were also physically apparent throughout the entire home, the parents realized the unintentional manifestation and wanted to make it better fast. After the consultation, the implemented adjustments shifted the household energetic patterns and therefore shifted how each person began to interact with the others. Typically, as everyone's chi gets accustomed to the changes, growing pains arise. Keep this in mind for yourself as you make adjustments in your own surroundings. An important part of the success in working on group issues under one household (or one office) is working through them together, increasing communication about why you are making these changes, and gaining input from all involved.

As you scan your home or office for positioning challenges, think about any struggles you might be having with your own ranking, title, status, importance, or personal perspective. Do you feel you are reaching your full potential? Do you feel in charge and in command of your career and relationships? First, the best way to embark upon tackling these challenges and more is by examining the physical position of three main pieces of your furniture over your lifetime. They are your bed, desk, and stove. When you think about the amount of time you are in position for sleeping, working, or cooking, it is reasonable to say that the position you are in for these three activities can then influence your psychological position for a good portion of your life. After examining these three mighty pillars and making the necessary adjustments, you can also begin to look at positioning in other areas of your home. A checklist at the end of the chapter will guide you.

Most people don't give much thought to the connection between how a piece of their furniture is located and how it can broaden a perspective, boost confidence, and facilitate goals. Picture this: You are seated at your desk at work. You are looking at the wall and your back is to the door. You cannot see who is entering or leaving. What is wrong with this position? An authoritative position is facing the door but not in direct alignment with it. David Daniel Kennedy, author of *Feng Shui for Dummies* (Hungry Minds, 2001), said it best when discussing position: "On a primordial level the evolutionary advantage goes to the person who is in a commanding position." By applying Feng Shui principles for arrangement, you can empower yourself to have an advantage—to not feel vulnerable and to feel more in charge. These boosts in empowerment—however subtle they may seem—can energetically affect your emotions and actions in a tremendous way.

DESK POSITIONING

The desk represents career and projects. The ideal desk position should be so that you are facing the door but not in direct alignment with it. Your back should be securely positioned against a wall and your view should be of the largest expanse of the room. If you are limited structurally and have no choice but to face the wall with your back or side to the door, hang a mirror—even a small one—with an adhesive backing. This can be placed on the top front surface of your computer. Or hang a mirror directly in front of you on the wall you are facing.

Having your desk positioned with your back to the door can create a feeling of vulnerability and continually put you at a disadvantage. Besides being easily startled, you can start to feel a loss of control in your life. At work, you might experience difficulties in being promoted, not being aware of inner workings of the company, and be more susceptible to being a victim of embezzlement or company subterfuge.

A client who worked from home was launching her own line of body products and wanted a consultation to help create an environment that supported her living and working goals. Right away, I noticed her back-to-the-door desk position. I was so sure she would feel a massive difference once it was moved that I suggested we reposition the desk right away. I had her sit down in the new position for a few moments to reconnect to her space from the new position of command. She liked it: "This feels totally different." I urge anyone who has their back to the door to turn around and face their world. Position yourself on a diagonal to the entrance if possible. If you don't believe that sitting in this position can evoke change for the better, I urge you to do the opposite. That's right. Put your desk facing the wall for at least nine days and see what happens. Notice how connected (or not) you feel to your surroundings. Observe any changes in your awareness when you are seated in this way.

A small-business owner had her desk situated so that she was head-to-head with her partner and had her back to the door. This position has the potential for pitting two people against each other. (A row of plants between the two can help deflect any opposition or tension that may occur.) One partner was in the commanding position while the other was not. Years passed, and their business, which consisted of two separate divisions, continued to flourish. However, one day the accountant informed them that an employee was stealing from one side of the company: the weaker positioned partner. The employee was confronted and let go, and the company continued to do well. The partner in the compromised desk position will have trouble seeing what is going on behind his or her back and be susceptible to or could even eventually partake in deception themselves.

If you are situated in an unfavorable position, it does not mean that your business is doomed to fail or you are about to engage in duplicitous business. What is certain is that there will be a potential for situations to occur where you "didn't see it coming" or felt you were not being as mindful to the business as you could have been. If this is your position, turn around, power up, and face the world.

Restricted Desk Options at Work

Many workplaces have a beige labyrinth of cubby configurations where temporary half-walls are erected and a feeling of bleakness pervades. If this is your situation, do all you can to make it your own, elevate your chi, and set yourself up to thrive. Repositioning your desk is hardly ever a realistic option in this situation, so focus more on the things you can change. Add a mirror in front of you so you can see who enters from behind. Make plants, such as ivy or snake plants (which are low-maintenance and even flourish under fluorescent lighting), an addition to your space, and invest in flowers as often as possible. Choose the pictures you display carefully. Don't display just any picture of your loved ones—choose the picture where the moment depicted is one that is truly uplifting. One client had a picture of her family on vacation displayed in her cubicle. When I asked about it, she revealed that the family was really stressed out in the picture. The glaring sun made them all look squinty, one of the kids was melting down, and she felt rushed to smile and pose. She loved her family. They made her feel good. But she didn't realize how the essence captured in that moment being displayed could add to her anxieties at work. Have you ever thought to examine the energy of the moment behind the pictures that you display? She later replaced the photograph with one where the posing wasn't forced and the feeling wasn't so stressed. She chose a funny moment where they were all secretly poking one another to make the others laugh. "I look at this picture every day, and I can't help but smile every single time. Whenever I am feeling job strain, I look at it and really feel lighter." It is often the little changes that add up to a considerable energetic shift in your space and, therefore, in yourself.

Positioning Yourself for Work Meetings

When seated in a room for a company meeting, the boss should be seated at the wealth area, which is the farthest, left corner from the door. Try to avoid seating yourself at the position directly in front of the door, with your back to the door. Often, people are drawn to the seat that they feel best represents their "placement" in the company. Clock-watchers tend to position themselves closest to the door. Notice if you have a tendency to be drawn to a particular seat, whether it's a company meeting or a restaurant. Where do you feel most comfortable? Do you let others decide where you will sit? This is perfectly acceptable when you are a guest in someone's home or out to lunch with a close friend. But when you need an edge—let's say you are feeling unsure, physically weak, or about to negotiate—be sure to choose the seat that will give you the best possible support.

IRENE: AN ADVANTAGE IN CORPORATE NEGOTIATIONS

Many corporations doing negotiations will never situate themselves with their backs to the door and will go to great lengths to have predetermined seating arranged beforehand. Irene worked for a Fortune 500 company as a company arbitrator dealing with unions. Irene describes the importance of positioning like this: "Company arbitrators always choose the seats with their backs to the windows, facing the door. We are fully aware of the psychological effects of positioning. It is a position of power and we always want to see who is coming and going at all times. This is true [securing the commanding position] despite the different venues we hold hearings in." They even go to great efforts to ensure that their seating is established in the commanding position beforehand. "Given the long history between the parties, it never seemed to be questioned where we would sit. To ensure that outcome, I or someone else in our team would get there early, survey the room, and put down pads and pens on 'our' side. We made sure we established that early on." Irene could not recall a time when they sat differently. And for results: "We won a majority of our hearings."

STOVE POSITIONING

The stove represents your finances and general health. The best position for it will allow the cook to face the main entrance to the room while cooking. It is important to keep the stove clean at all times and make sure the area around it is well lit and that all burners function properly. Be certain that you are using all of your burners and not favoring just one. You can ensure this by rotating your teakettle from burner to burner with each use.

JENNY: A JOURNEY THROUGH POSITIONING

Jenny was renovating a newly purchased home and told me that she was clashing with her architect every time she wanted to make changes in the plans or materials. She told me that her stove had become a point of contention. The architect preferred it on an island, which would have put it in the commanding position because the cook would be facing the wide entryway to the kitchen. Jenny and the interior designer wanted it on what they called "the focal point wall." After Jenny saw two of her new neighbors' homes, she told me she felt compelled to make even more changes to "keep up with the block." It was important to Jenny to have a statement wall with intricate stonework and a large hood over the double stove. She called me in to look at the architect's renderings and lend my perspective. I explained to her how the stove represents your well-being and finances. I reinforced the architect's vision and made my case using perspectives stemming from aesthetic, function, and even venerable wisdom. It did not work. Jenny would not budge. Jenny was set on a "grand setting," and her vision of a dramatic statement wall needed the stove on it.

Months later, Jenny contacted me and said because "the economy had taken a turn for the worse," she was financially unable to keep up with her profligate renovations. She was about to sell the house and was consumed with how her peers would view her. Throughout the renovation process, Jenny was fixated on position in numerous definitions of the word. Literally, her resolute stance on the stove position was unwavering and superficially based. Metaphorically, her perceived position (or status) in society was an overriding concern behind most of her decisions.

If Jenny had not run out of money and kept the stove where she preferred, chances are her obsession with status would increase because this fixation would have been reinforced even more so in her home from the groundwork up. Her change in finances offered an opportunity to step back and observe her motivations and reflect on the life she was creating. It was a lengthy and intense process in working with Jenny (two more homes, a mastectomy, and a divorce) to get to a place where she finally felt she was living authentically, within her means, and as she described, "living a bit humbler, a bit happier."

I find so many of the ancient principles to intuitively feel logical. However, with the many different schools of Feng Shui that have evolved over thousands of years, there are several interpretations that have a strong basis in superstition. Most of their superstitious tenets are fear-based. That is where you will hear things like "Don't position a mirror in the bedroom or it will steal your soul!" I personally find it irrational and don't operate from a point of credulous fear. It disturbs me that this is even out there representing Feng Shui. It's not empowering nor does it lead to success and happiness because you are basing your decisions on being afraid. That is why, after years and years of study, research, and client consultations, I've learned to take the parts that deliver reasonable logic and are proven to work, toss or update the ones that don't, use a dose of intuition, and bring it all together with mind, body, and spirit connections. It's a formula that works for my clients and myself and will work for you, too.

Stove Positioning Tips

According to age-old Chinese lore, stove positioning is important. This means avoiding "startled chi" by having the cook face the door while at the stove and not surprised by people coming from behind. To me, it's common sense to situate yourself like this—not only at the stove but for the bed and desk, too, to give yourself a subconscious boost so you feel more prepared and strengthened—even if the effects might feel barely imperceptible to you. If this position is unavoidable, a brass wind chime or a bamboo flute hung above is the classic Feng Shui recommendation to redirect the energy and offer protection for the cook. Since this decorative addition may not work for most, I might suggest a reflective tile backsplash. In traditional Feng Shui, it's believed that prosperity for the household will occur if the cook can stand at the stove and look to the center of the house.

Realistically, relocating a stove is not an easy structural task for most. When I am consulting on large luxury high-rises for developers who require a modern Feng Shui solution but cannot move the stove to its power spot, I offer up other solutions, like the reflective backsplash.

When given the choice, natural gas burning stoves are better than electric stoves even when considering air quality issues. The fire that gas stoves generates is more organic, closer to the Fire Element in its pure form, and produces less electrical magnetic fields.

From a holistic perspective, the stove represents the epicenter of the household because it is the maker of sustenance and the conduit to health and wellness, and therefore is our lifeline in our ability to create wealth. Keep it clean at all times.

Bed Positioning

Your bed represents marriage, relationships, and general success. You should be positioned in the farthest corner away from the door so that while lying in bed you can see the door but you are not in direct alignment with it (bed position 1, 2, or 3 on page 119). The bed should be up against a non-bathroom wall with space to walk around the three sides of the bed. The reason you should not place your bed against a bathroom wall is because you do not want to have your head alongside such active energy. Bathrooms represent constant movement and riddance with flushing, running water, and drains. The frequent movement of the plumbing system, both literally and symbolically, are not conducive to good health. The same goes for facing a bathroom while lying in bed. If this position cannot be avoided, always make sure you keep the bathroom door closed. Avoid putting a bed directly under a window because it diminishes support. However, if this is your only structural option, try to create a feeling of solidity behind your bed with a sturdy headboard or curtains that can be closed at night to keep out the active chi (light, wind, noise, etc.).

Chinese folklore teaches us not to position your bed so that your feet are directly in line with the door. This is considered the "coffin position." Regardless of the primeval philosophy, having your bed positioned in this way (or even in position 4,

BED POSITIONING RECOMMENDATIONS

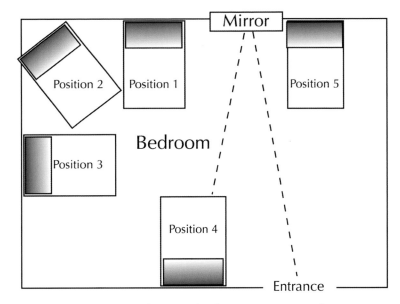

Bed placement 1, 2, and 3 are the best positions. If position 4 is your only option, hang a mirror that enables you to see who is entering the room. Avoid position 5 because it is in straight alignment with the door and the direct line of chi will make sleeping difficult.

as long as you don't have a beautiful view opposite the entrance) innately does not feel right for the majority of people. It simply makes sense to choose position 1, 2, or 3 if you have your choice.

The holistic connections to your bed are just as significant. When you are sleeping, you are at your most vulnerable. Your body is rejuvenating, growing, and healing on a cellular and subconscious level. You are most susceptible to the energies of your environment while in this state, which makes positioning the bed crucial. If you are lying in your bed and you cannot see the door to your bedroom, try to reposition your bed in a more empowering position. If you are limited structurally, then a mirror can be hung on the opposite wall to strengthen your position, enabling you to see who is entering (bed position 4).

During a consultation, a client showed me an extra bedroom in the basement that was occasionally used by a relative. The unmade bed in the center of the room was without a headboard. Without being flush against a wall, the bed was floating in the center of the room. A floating bed is like a sailboat lost at sea without a sail. With a bed in this state, whoever slept there would surely be off course and in troubled relationship waters. In this scenario, that was the case. The person sleeping there was in the midst of an unconventional and troubled relationship and was described by the homeowner as being in limbo, just like the bed appeared to be. Beds floating in the center of a room rarely work well.

Positioning Tips for Home, Office, and the Classroom at Home

Look at your kitchen and dining tables. Who sits where? Does everyone have a designated spot? This is recommended to bring a sense of consistency and reliability to family dining. But if you feel your family is stuck in a rut, then switch up seating to gain a fresh perspective. Gathering nightly for family meals around the dinner table is crucial in building a sense of cohesiveness and harmony.

When having a sit-down dinner party, a round table is the first choice and makes for a better conversational flow. Next choice is a narrower, rectangular dining table. If you are more than three feet apart from the person across from you, you will be straining to connect and conversation will be limited. When in your own home, always situate your guests at the commanding position.

Avoid positioning a child's or teenager's bed under windows. The chi is too active and can lead to restless sleep and concentration problems.

In an Office

Choose the wealth position on the floor plan for your office if you have the option to do so. If not, make sure that within your own office you position your desk so you face out toward the door but are not in direct alignment with it. Choose this far left position for chair placement in meetings as well. If you are sitting in a cubicle,

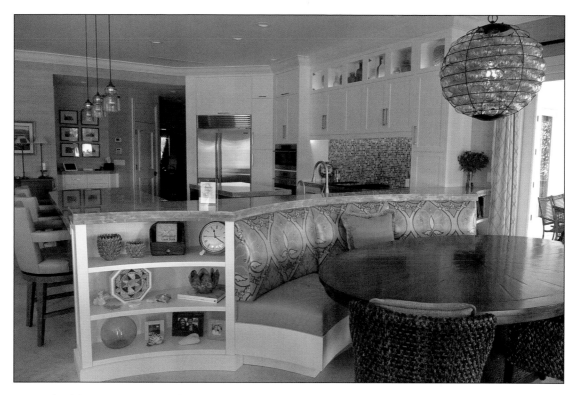

Round tables are more conducive to balanced conversation.

adhere a mirror in front of you, or at the top of your computer, so you can see behind you.

In the Classroom

Securing the best position in the classroom is essential in gaining the most you can from the curriculum, particularly in working with your own learning style. Generally, in a row formation, sitting from mid to front row is best. Being situated closest to the door can create a strong itch to leave, so students who do not have a propensity to bolt early should be situated there. Gathering desks together in small groups works best for elementary school classrooms. Student desks should not be facing out toward windows or hallways. They should be turned toward the teacher.

SANDRA: A ROLE OF RESPONSIBILITY

Sandra was showing me her beautiful, open-air island home in Maui. She was quite frustrated with her husband's recreational drug use, which had escalated from an occasional indulgence to a daily, destructive habit. She was carrying the responsibility of the family in every way for nearly twenty years and was feeling weary. When we got to her bedroom, I knew immediately which side she slept on without even asking her. The double bed was positioned so that one person in the bed was in direct alignment with the bedroom door—receiving an undeviating line of nonstop, rushing chi—and that was Sandra. Her position paralleled her role in the family. She was the one who took the most upon herself to support the household—financially, emotionally, and physically.

I encouraged her to switch sides of the bed with her husband and warned her to proceed with caution. She was ready to switch and felt hopeful that it would encourage things to get better between them. When I followed up weeks later, she said that he refused to do that because "he likes his position and does not want to change." I offered secondary recommendations that involved ways to strengthen Sandra's chi independently at first, without upsetting the invariable and volatile frame of mind of her husband. This process is more like running a Crock-Pot on low for several hours. Eventually it gets the job done, but it's not a quick fire. I had her move the entire bed as much as possible out of the direct alignment from the bedroom entrance. (Which ended up being only about two feet over because of the structural layout of the room.) Her husband still kept "his" position, but this enabled Sandra to recharge and take less of an energetic hit. I asked Sandra to choose ways outside of the house that would always position her in a commanding manner. I encouraged her to cultivate her chi through meditation and to begin to put herself first. When only one partner in a marriage is making necessary changes for the better, sooner or later the other will hopefully adjust to the new chi or the marriage will endure more conflict. I don't know the outcome with Sandra and her husband. Her email changed and we lost touch.

Transformations are obviously most probable when the person is open to change or at least aware that a modification could be beneficial. Sandra's husband was not ready for change and feared an alteration is his routine. Whenever fear enters, it holds those back from making a difference in their lives, which could allow the best to unfold. Any decision made from fear-based thinking is never a good one. The hopeful thinkers look at change as a source of inspiration and growth. Fearful thinkers are threatened by change because of the unknown possibilities based in insecurity or losing control. It is essential to know that once you trust in the Universe and make your decisions from a position of empowered thinking and pure intention, then your divine path can open out with rich lessons to embrace. If we don't change and reflect, we don't grow.

By creating positions in your home that facilitate your goals—such as relaxation in this spot above—you are allowing them to happen more easily.

HOLISTIC POSITIONING CHECKLIST

Mind: Try to reflect on all the various meanings of the positions in your life. Think of all your roles. Maybe you are a wife, activist, CEO, volunteer, writer, cook. Look closely at how these roles may be showing up in your space in ways that need improvement.

Body: Think of the actions that you take that are related to these roles or positions in your life. For example, as a tired working mom at the end of the day, are you plunging into a bed that is set up for support? As a daring entrepreneur, are you stacking odds in your favor by arranging your desk properly? Make sure that you are setting yourself up to embrace change when necessary and are empowering yourself to get in position to take command and rule your world!

Spirit: As you reflect on your positions in the world and your physical positioning in your home, try to draw the connections to where possible challenges may be residing. When you take an action to adjust yourself into a more commanding position, dovetail that action with a detailed visualization of how this new perspective is strengthening and supporting you. Envision a specific, positive outcome. Know that energetically you are creating an atmosphere that is supporting your soul's desires. Ask yourself, how does your position of your spirituality affect you on a daily basis? How are you tapping into your faith to help guide you in all areas of your life? Is it a part of the joys, or only there when you are grieving, ill, or in need? The more you can add your own religion or the essence of your own spirituality into everything you do, from your perspective on life to the setup of your space, the more full and meaningful your life will be.

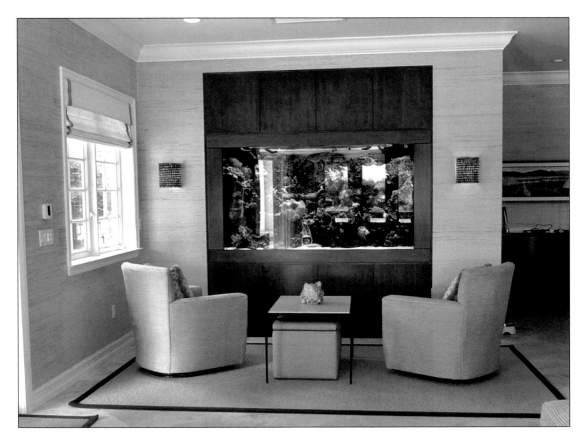

When you create an intentional space for your goals—like relaxation here—it is easier to achieve them.

A space that is thoughtfully positioned for success challenges you to examine your life more wholly. This will make your space feel more comforting, supportive, and functional. You will feel more aware and present in your space and connected in your life. By exploring position holistically in every sense of the word, from the physical (your bed, desk, and stove) to the mental (perspective, roles, and titles) and adding in your spiritual beliefs, your challenges and setbacks can be handled more easily and in a complete way.

CHAPTER SIX

Yin and Yang: Finding Your Balance

Change is the nature of the universe.

—*I Ching*, "The Book of Change"

George was thirty-eight years old and a bachelor. He lived by himself in a modest one-bedroom condominium in a suburban town and worked as a computer programmer. After twenty years of casually dating various women, he felt ready for a serious relationship and hoped to get married and have children. He tried Internet dating, speed dating, and blind dating and was feeling discouraged with the results. He emailed me for a consultation and sent pictures of his place. Every picture revealed a sterile-looking environment with sharp edges, straight lines, bright lighting, and bold geometric patterns. Basically, every detail I saw represented Yang expressions.

When there is a dominance of one force over another, an imbalance will inevitably occur. Yin and Yang are the Chinese perspective of balance and continual change. These forces divide everything in the universe into two categories. The female, dark colors, soft seating, dim lighting, quiet rooms like bedrooms and bathrooms represent Yin. The male, bright lighting, large spaces, bold geometric patterns, and active rooms such as laundry, kitchen, and family rooms represent Yang. This profound theory views opposites as evolving and cycling forces that govern the Universe. There is neither a right nor a wrong, but there is balance, transformation, and interaction. A duality cannot exist without both parts, which then mutually create a balance.

It is common for me to feel my strongest intuitive sense of a space when I first walk through the client's door. I can rely on this to happen fairly often. Once in George's home, I didn't feel entirely comfortable. My discomfort was not directed at George—he was a kind and hospitable man, immediately taking my coat and offering me a beverage. I sat down on a straight-backed, hard metal chair and tried to get comfortable. I looked around. I was hard pressed to find a single item that represented a softer, darker, feminine Yin side. The coffee table was glass and had a jagged pattern, collections were minimal, lighting was very bright, wall colors were all white, and artwork was large geometric designs in bold primary colors. George had moved in almost a year ago.

After chatting for a few minutes, I asked him, "What have any of the women you have dated thought about your place?"

"A couple times I have had some women over for dinner and all, but I would have to say that I tend to spend more time at their home or traveling to other places together for a weekend . . . but it's been a while."

After walking through George's home, we came back to the living room, and I explained the Tao and the Yin and Yang theory and pointed out all of the Yang energy that surrounded him—from hard edges to bold artwork. There was a vital imbalance in the opposing forces of Yin and Yang that needed to be tweaked in his home. Since George was trying to bring feminine energy into his life, it was crucial that he first start right in his home. "All we need to do is turn up the volume on the Yin around here," I assured George.

George admitted he was awkward around interior design matters and would not know where to start. I asked him to take me to his necktie collection and show me his favorite tie. He pulled out a tie with a small paisley print in dark blue, hunter green, and rust colors. I based most of my Yin interior design suggestions around that tie. I told him to bring his tie with him as the source of inspiration when he shopped or keep it near him if he would be purchasing online. By bringing in some softness, rounded corners, plush cushions, warmer colors, and light dimmers, he would quickly feel a difference. A good place to begin was with some bed linens and pillows. I recommended that he start with a cozy chenille or cashmere throw, down-filled plush pillows for the couch, and the highest thread count sheets that he could afford, all the while referring back to his tie as the inspirational color palette. It wasn't a difficult strategy.

"If floral artwork is too feminine for you, look for seductive images or landscapes with smooth, soft lines. Add fresh flowers. Buy candles and light them regularly. Plants should be supple with rounded leaves, not aloe or cacti." He took notes.

Even his music was all Yang—only hard rock—so I recommended he add some mellower tunes to his playlist to create a different atmosphere, yet still have the soul and funky beat that he liked. I wanted to assure him that tapping into this "foreign" force did not mean that he would lose his masculinity—only enhance it by adding another facet to complement it. Yin and Yang need each other. The same advice of adding the missing Yang energy would be given to either a male or female living in a predominately Yin atmosphere.

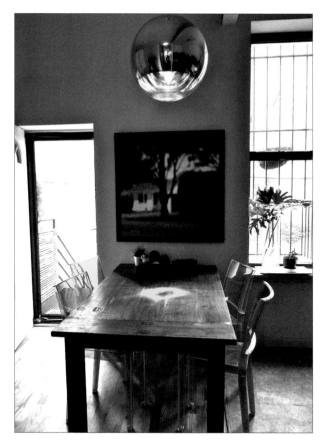

The framed picture of a sports car, the calendar of bikini models, and the dartboard in his living room were removed, and George said he would replace them with "things that bring out my softer side." I could see that he had the desire to complete this project, and he would discover a lot about himself in the meantime.

As I left, I said, "Nothing is a hundred percent Yin or a hundred

Mixing old and new is a great way to create a Yin and Yang balance.

percent Yang. You need the Yin to know the Yang and vice versa. You just needed a little direction, but you are already on your way." George kept me updated on the changes in his apartment via lots of email pictures, and I was pleased at how he took on the recommendations with such verve and individuality. His place completely transformed from hapless Yang bachelor pad to a cozy, warm, and inviting abode. His love life blossomed too. He told me he met his new girlfriend while shopping for bed linens!

TRISHA: A BACHELOR PAD FOR THE FAMILY

In Trisha's bio, I was stuck on the sentence, "I can't be in my bedroom alone." Reading that bothered me, but not as much as when I was actually in her bedroom for the consultation and felt extremely uneasy and vulnerable myself. I was standing in a large room with thirty-foot ceilings. One wall had an ominous skyline mural that was spread over an entire wall. It pictured a dark, indefinable city landscape in black, gray, and white. The two main pieces of furniture in the room were a king-size bed with a custom-built eighteen-foot headboard console made of a shiny gray lacquer and a matching gargantuan gray armoire that housed shelving and a large-screen television. The giant pieces, situated in such a lofty and expansive room, made one feel like a child, playing in a disproportionately large-scale playhouse. I felt lost and insignificant standing in the space. The occupants bought the house completely furnished five years prior and found it to be cold, sterile, and uncomfortable, and now called me in for help.

While in the bedroom, I had a hard time shaking the energy of the previous owner. "How would you describe the man who previously owned your home?" I asked.

"He was cold, aloof—not warm," she said. Her description of his demeanor nearly matched her own description of the home that she purchased from him and didn't yet make her own. (Not surprising. Notice how you describe someone and then try to describe his or her home. Often there are parallels or same word descriptions that cross over. More on this in the next chapter.) Being that they bought the house completely furnished, it caused the lingering predecessor energy to remain even stronger over the years. The previous owner was described as a hard-partying bachelor, and every room emanated his Yang energy. It was physically showcased in the oversize bar that sat eight and took center stage of the house, in the enormous metal front doors, and in the severe angular shapes of the home's exterior and interior. The client was warm, compassionate, and loving toward others—especially to her two young children. Her gentle, loving Yin energy radiated around her and was being cut, conflicted, and stunted by the Palace of Yang that she lived in. It was obvious that her priorities were her children; both of their rooms were thoughtfully redecorated and perfectly suitable for their growing spirits.

The rest of the house needed softening. The simple solutions, just like in George's consultation, included adding plants, flowers, comfortable throws, cushy pillows, and texturized rugs. The medium tasks involved painting a significant amount of the walls with warmer tones. The more advanced suggestions involved replacing the heavy, large metal front doors with wood ones, adding more wood furniture and accessories, and using the color green and warm earth tones throughout the home. Instead of white, bright walls, the vast space called for warmer colors. I urged most of the previous homeowner's furniture to be given to charity, passed on, or sold, and doing so should be accompanied by the vision that all the negative predecessor energy was leaving the house as well.

Perhaps it wouldn't be a "balanced" chapter without a preponderating Yin story, but I have not had a consultation that was completely dominated by Yin forces! There certainly have been spaces where Yin aspects were present, but if there was a strictly extreme Yin situation, it might look something like this: A small, dimly lit home with low ceilings that was overcrowded and cluttered with knickknacks, dark walls, and floral or intricate patterns. Occupants would most likely feel inactive, lethargic, depressed, and submissive to whatever challenges life happens to throw at them. The location of the house might be near a cemetery or church where there are a lot of funerals. A home that is dominantly Yin can feel heavy and run down.

Holistic Tips to Elevate the Space of a Yin Environment

Yin extreme spaces can feel dark, heavy, and depressed.

Mind

Create routines that inspire action. Instead of automatically turning on the television, reach for music and play upbeat tunes that make you want to dance or sing.

Tend to all repairs as soon as you possibly can. An ongoing list of unfinished projects subconsciously diminishes your energy.

Body

Increase wattage in all bulbs throughout the house. Use the "natural light" bulbs that reveal the full spectrum of colors in their intended glory.

If the outside view is pleasant, try to bring it in as much as possible by using mirrors that reflect the outside scenery.

Position chairs to be located near windows.

Add plenty of life force, for example, pets, live plants, and flowers. Invest in an air purifier that moves and cleans the stagnant air.

Spirit

Use aromatherapy to tap into the spiritual essence of each essential oil. Choose a scent like lemon, grapefruit, neroli, sweet orange, or bergamot, which has been proven in studies to uplift spirits.

Holistic Tips to Decrease the Yang Energy of an Overactive Space

Sometimes overactive homes or offices have too much Yang energy and can lead to aggression, anger, and burn out.

Mind

Replace red, orange, and yellow with calmer tones of blues, greens, and beige.

Examine the message of imagery in your surroundings. Replace fast-moving images (sports cars, mobiles, cheetahs, etc.) with images or items that cause you to stop and reflect (water fountains, pictures that inspire stillness, interesting plants and flowers).

Body

Cover all clear glass tabletops with a runner or tablecloth. Add a centerpiece that is also a conversational piece, and make sure dining chairs are not hard and sleek but are cushy and comfortable. This leads to lingering over meals longer than you ordinarily would. Family dinners will not seem as hurried, and dinner parties will feel more engaging.

Add additional rugs to large expanses of open space.

Spirit

Add heavy objects to symbolically anchor the chi, such as a statue, large rock, or sculpture.

Every room of the house can be divided into a Yin or a Yang room based on the activities that occur there. Active rooms include foyer, living room, family room, kitchen, playroom, laundry room, and garage. Areas where relaxation, contemplation, sleeping, or minimal activity occur are considered Yin rooms. They are dens, bedrooms, storage areas, basements, and bathrooms.

Yin and Yang of the Room		
	Yin	**Yang**
Room Size	Small	Large
Location in the House	Quiet, Private	Noisy, Busy
Room's View	Intimate	Grand
Ceiling	Low	High
Natural Light	Low	Bright
Electric Light	Dim	Bright
Open Floor Space	Small Amounts	Large Expanses
Floors	Dark or Ornate	Light or Plain
Wall Colors	Medium, Dark, or Muted	Light or Bright
Furniture	Many Pieces	Few Pieces
Furniture Colors	Dark	Light or Bright
Furniture and Décor	Small and Low	Large and High
Seating	Soft and Padded	Hard, Unpadded
Furniture Shapes	Curved, Rounded Lines	Straight, Angular Lines
Patterns	Floral	Geometric
Fabrics	Textured	Smooth and Shiny
Design	Elaborate, Layered, Ornate	Plain, Uncomplicated
Displayed Collections	Many	Few or None
Art	Many Small Pieces	Large or Few Pieces
Pillows	Many	Few or None
Books	Many	Few or None
Mirrors	Small	Large
Plants	Many	Few or None

Go through the table on the previous page and notice what forces dominate your home. Ideally we want an even balance; however, some rooms need to be more Yin dominant, and others need to be more Yang. Remember that within Yin there is Yang and vice versa—one cannot exist without the other. If you have an extreme uneven equilibrium of the two, chances are you will be experiencing a Yin/Yang imbalance in some way in your life as well.

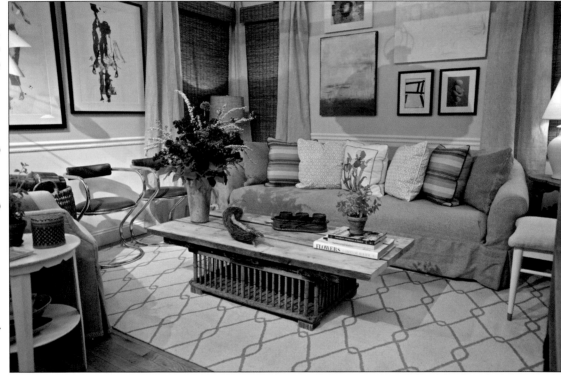

Courtesy of Keita Turner Design and Edgar Scott Photography.

This living room has a sensible blend of Yin and Yang attributes, which creates a balanced energy.

MY STORY: HARNESSING THESE EVER-EVOLVING FORCES

I'm a Gemini. So I was innately born with a duality that can vacillate quite easily from minute to minute or day to day. I often reflect on certain phases in my life that were so Yang, such as leaving a solid and prosperous career in New York to move to

Maui alone, getting a motorcycle, and training as a stuntwoman while I sold radio commercials and sarongs (two separate jobs). Then I think about where I am now. My stable, Yin-filled life as a nurturing mom and wife, preferring to stay in all day, cook, write, and make anything creative. I can't imagine taking risks now in my forties like I did in my twenties, and I am quite content with that. However, my career now forces me to Yang it up in order to subsist, and my role as a mother and wife encourages me to sometimes take action out of my comfort zone I wouldn't necessarily choose. (Thankfully—otherwise I'm sure I'd turn into a crazy-crafting-sloth-hermit.)

Life is a constant ebb and flow in many ways. Sometimes predominant Yang periods must occur, such as action, creation, or conflict. Other times contemplation, destruction, or silence is necessary. There are no absolutes, and each force is dependent upon the other to evolve and transform. When a cycle of preponderate Yin or Yang runs its course, it is important to pause and reflect in order to extract the lessons from that influence. If there is no cessation and a singular force, for example Yang, overrides your life, then—burnout, rock bottom, exhaustion. We have all heard about the necessity of balance in life to the point of it sounding rote. Really understanding this concept is about utilizing opposing forces to harness the best of each force—for whatever moment you are in, cycle of your life you are dealing with, conversation you are engaged in—so that you can fully experience life more deeply and equalized.

My husband, John, is an extremely active, take-charge, manly man with a thundering voice and a core so steadfast in goodness you can feel his purity of heart in every conversation. While his external energies may appear very Yang with his masculine, sometimes unrefined traits, his internal predisposition is quite Yin. He is not a man with an overblown ego; doesn't care if another is "stealing his spotlight" or cutting him off in traffic. His steadfast, calm internal demeanor and ability to not respond so reactively, I assume, also helps him in navigating high-adrenaline situations that he endures as a captain in the FDNY. His left brain dominates with logic, reason, and analytical thinking.

Our daughter, Luchia, has gathered and personalized what I feel is the best of both Yin and Yang forces within the two of us. She recently finished her first kids' triathlon, and, on a regular basis, she is engaged in an active lifestyle (biking, skiing, skateboarding, inline skating, hiking, and *all* sports) with her father and experiences more cerebral, spiritual, creative, or indoor activities with me. In her third-grade Identity Study at school, she said, in part, "To you I am a girl with long hair and skirts who does ballet. But to me, I am also a good soccer player, a great skier and I can get my hands dirty. I am not a girly girl, although I can be at times. I am unique, quirky, funny, and creative . . . I am a helping hand that will give to others . . . I am a survivor." I have no doubt that the balance of our predominant energies blended together has enabled our offspring to recognize and utilize these forces within herself in order to fully experience the benefits of both.

My husband and I are comfortable in our roles as partners, yet we have benefited significantly from the opposing energetic lessons we have learned from each other.

We see the value in each other's Yin and Yang attributes and have respect and admiration for them. I asked John what lessons my soul has taught him, and he answered, "Laura's soul has taught me to try to understand the spiritual side of life. The life force that stays alive after we are gone or the life force that tries to come back and touch the living. The deep connection we have to all other spiritual life forces that exist. I do not understand it all but am trying to, I guess that's why it takes a lifetime. In the end I know her soul is preparing me for what lays ahead tomorrow, next month, and eventually the end."

When I reflect on my soul lessons in this lifetime, there is a profound internal undercurrent of Yang that resides in the depth of my overactive, over-proliferating bone marrow. Yang forces continue on right up to my surface with reactions that are quick to present when buttons are pressed or when patience is needed. Internal restraint in these regards feel like my elusive life goal for big-picture balance. Meanwhile, as is quite common with many couples, my chosen life partner is the energetic internal counterbalance. He is there, internally peaceful and patient, leading by example. While I haven't figured out how to naturally slow down my bone marrow, it is up to me to shift my perspective of ego-ingrained behaviors and inherent reactions. Using Yin and Yang for the checks and balances of life is a surefire way to help me with that.

YIN AND YANG LESSONS OF THE SOUL IN PARTNERSHIPS

Whether loving partnerships are male and female, male and male, or female and female, it doesn't mean that the male in the relationship is the Yang and the female is the Yin. It is the predominate energies themselves that make that designation, and even that can change at times throughout one's life. From previous relationships to current ones, it can be revealing to reflect on how Yin and Yang energies have been in excess, absent, or generally balanced in your life. When there have been imbalances, was there a lot of conflict, silence, or separation? Were your relationships mostly balanced but the relationship itself ran its course? If you are someone who is shy, reflective, or slow to react (all Yin qualities), has your partner added to those qualities or encouraged you to get out of your comfort zone? Are you hot-tempered and your partner knows how to cool you down? The cultivation of recognizing the pros and cons within your partner can make your appreciation for each other that much deeper.

If you don't have a Yin/Yang balance, it doesn't mean that your partnership is doomed. It means that there are other lessons going on there, but you could most likely benefit from bringing in some opposing forces. There certainly can be two Yangs dominating the world in Type A fashion (however, that could mean a lot of ongoing competition, clashes, and unrest that govern the relationship), and just like night is to day, a sense of equilibrium is necessary for healthy and stable relationships. Some people will deeply carry their negative Yang or Yin personality traits into relationship after relationship. Breaking the negative pattern of excess can be tough to do—especially if the truth of their Yin or Yang propensity is not being honestly acknowledged. This brings up the question: what can you do if your live-in partner cannot recognize his or her Yin/Yang shortcomings? If your relationship feels out of balance, look to bring the opposing energy into the space. While going through your home, ask yourself how the Yin and Yang energies are present or absent. How do they enhance or diminish the negative traits of your partner? Depending upon the depth of their denial, sometimes adjusting the opposing force can make the imbalanced partner feel ill at ease and opposed to the exact energy that is necessary to foster his or her own growth. When that occurs, it's best to integrate those needed forces in small doses. You can also use the Feng Shui bagua map to enhance not only your relationships, but many other areas of your life as well.

YIN AND YANG TIPS THROUGHOUT THE BAGUA

When going through the bagua map of your home, keep in mind that both forces are needed, and each energy has its vital place in different phases of your life just as much as it does in the different rooms of your home.

Family

This section of the bagua should aim for equal male/female energy. The Yin aspects should feel warm and nurturing. The Yang forces should feel motivating. An example might be to add Wood, such as plants, which is a nurturing element (Yin), and increase lighting (Yang).

Wealth

Add Yin aspects when you need to sustain your wealth, Yang when you wish to control or activate it. In the wealth area, a heavy objet d'art will enhance the Yin forces to stabilize wealth flow; chimes will help activate the energy.

Health

In traditional Chinese medicine, it is believed that the imbalance of Yin and Yang are the basis for disease. Homeostasis requires the avoidance of extremes. Yang in excess makes Yin suffer, while Yin in excess makes Yang suffer. If you are suffering from a Yang condition where organs are overactive or heat is excessive (overactive bladder, over proliferation of blood cells, heat stroke), try to add more Yin conditions to your living space. Do the opposite for Yin health conditions by adding Yang energy.

Career

To lead or follow. To begin or end. To listen or speak. Each valid Yin or Yang decision changes from moment to moment throughout a career path. The key is to know when to make use of each choice at the appropriate time or when to employ both. A new mother stopped her Wall Street job to raise her child and found she had days when she was missing the daily interaction of her peers and the action of an office environment. When she experienced those feelings, she said she only had to look into the eyes of her child and realize that she was doing the most important work of her life, right now, at this moment. Sometimes when we feel like we are in an extreme phase of our professional life (such as being laid off or, conversely, working extra hours) we must remind ourselves of the balance that can live within, like an inner compass guiding us to the next destined cycle. Each phase is rich in experiences that help us with the next succession in our existence. We just have to strive to figure it out and acknowledge it when we are in the moment.

Helpful People & Travel

This gua is the embodiment of both Yin and Yang powers. Supportive, compassionate "helpers" in our life enhance the essence of Yin. Actively seeking, exploring, and traveling are all Yang energies. Try to reflect that equality of energy in this area of your home.

Children & Creativity

Creative energy is Yang. Receiving energy is Yin. In order to create, we must be receptive to receive inspiration. Enhance creative energies by tapping into your own male/female aspects. If you are experiencing a creative block, allow yourself to take an action that will encourage receiving. This might be going for a run, listening to music, or going to a museum.

Children's rooms should emanate more Yin than Yang. Their bedrooms should be a soothing oasis promoting safety and calmness. Keep Yang visuals (bold reds and blues or vehicle themes) to other play areas.

Knowledge & Spirituality

Mental exertion is Yin and physical performance is Yang. Yoga is a great example of unifying mind with body to achieve both spiritual and physical wellness. But any activity (Yang) where you find "mindfulness" (Yin), such as taking a quiet walk or even making your tea, can be an opportunity to enhance your own spiritual path.

Relationship

We all have both forces of Yin and Yang blended within ourselves. When you are in a healthy relationship, most likely your dominating force is complementary to your mate's latent one. The journey of aiding a mate to develop hidden opposing energies can be fulfilling and quite fun.

YIN AND YANG WITHIN YOURSELF: CREATING AN INTERNAL BALANCE BY EXAMINING YOUR HOME

The quiet, shy, inwardly focused personality is labeled as Yin dominant, and the extroverted, assertive, aggressive type is Yang. But we know that we are all complex beings that can go through changes, moods, phases, and moments when we operate in either force at different times. The key is to discover your general personality propensity while also looking into the predominant force that resides in your home.

If your personality is Yin dominate, is your home also set up that way? If it is, you'll find it harder to get out of your comfort zone when needed. If you tend to be impulsive, overly talkative, or an adrenaline junkie, is your home counterbalancing that with Yin forces or enhancing that more with Yang ones? Next, honestly assess when Yin or Yang behaviors are not working for you. If you find yourself always in the role of giver, you'll end up being exhausted or resentful unless you start allowing some receiving to happen. You can instigate this goal—or any others—by adding more design elements of the opposing force into your home. This is the physical, or body, portion of holistically addressing this issue.

Next, challenge yourself by forcing yourself to take on the opposing trait from what you would normally do. This is the mental or the mind part. When friends and family get together, are you the one that does all the talking? Make a point of really listening—not thinking about other things or what you are going to say next—just focus on listening and asking thoughtful questions. Is it hard for you to make a decision quickly? When that happens again, try checking in with your gut and just going for it.

What is important to understand about Yin and Yang is that throughout your life, you are continuously going through phases, cycles, moments, and situations where there is more Yin, less Yang needed and vice versa. Similar to a balanced relationship, there is a give and take that sustains the dance of a mutually meaningful interaction. This is the spiritual part. There is a sense of grounding that occurs when your relationship feels solid because of complementary forces between you. There can be greater health if there is an internal and external balance between action (exercise, healthy choices) and inaction (meditation, rest). Now you hold the key to knowing when to ignite the fire or control the flame within yourself, your relationships, your goals, your health, and your surroundings.

CHAPTER SEVEN

Living with Intention: Creating a Home with Soul

"By tapping into our inner gifts and living each day in alignment with our best, worthiest, most honorable intentions, we'll find our path through the world."

—Mallika Chopra, *Living With Intent*

Imagine your basic economy motel room with standard matching furniture, television, and some lackluster framed prints on the wall. This is an example of a space without soul. But that's okay (for the most part), because budget motel rooms aim to keep personality and personalization out of it to accommodate all the travelers laying their temporary claim. This motel room is an extreme example in order to familiarize you with a space void of depth, atmosphere, and personality, but there are also fully decorated homes with permanent residents that can feel soulless. Imagine a brand new spec home that is staged for an open house or a strategically positioned room in a furniture catalog where everything is only from that one store. These spaces may suit their purpose perfectly fine, but they deliver examples of spaces that lack soul.

A home with soul can feel like a warm hug—much like eating a home-cooked meal made with love. Whenever the judges on the television show *Top Chef* had contestant Carla Hall's food, they'd nearly always say that her food "had soul and was made with love." Hall defined her philosophy of "cooking with love" as putting one's own care and warmth into food. She believes that if one is happy and calm while

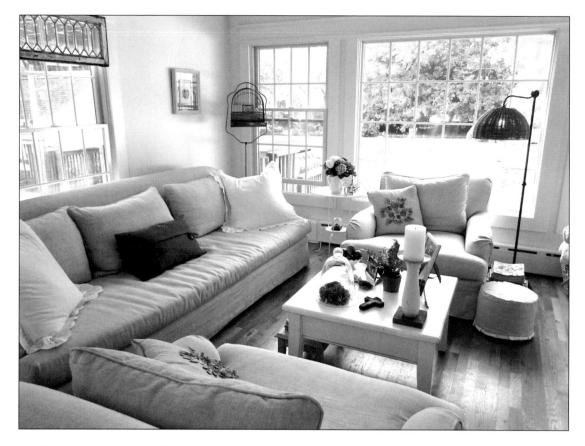

cooking, then this will show in the food, making it much better, whereas if one feels otherwise, it will degrade their cuisine. The same is true for your home. It takes care and warmth—as well as thoughtful decisions—to create a happy home with soul.

This chapter reveals how your own "soul" can manifest in your space by your decorating choices, by making sure your own voice is being heard, and by not letting fear take over.

DECORATING STYLES: WHAT OUR CHOICES MAY REVEAL

With the first glance at the interior design of the intimate surroundings we call home, our tastes and lifestyles can be revealed. When we look deeper and draw the holistic connections, we can better understand our own emotional and psychological interiors and discover what our desires, motivations, fears, or challenges might be. Our interior design choices are really a self-actualization expedition. This discovery of self and interconnectedness begins right in your own living room.

A formula for an inviting living room like this one: plenty of comfortable seating, interesting gathered objects, live plants or flowers, lighting options ranging from task to dimmable, a variety of textures, meaningful art, a focal point or place for the eye to rest, and general tidiness!

We all have certain ideas and conceptions attached to interior design styles. It may not be a stretch to imagine the personality traits of one who lives in a grand and opulent baroque style home as someone who might have a magnanimous ego or has reached some financial success or is at least *trying* to portray that. Someone who lives in a home that is void of style or character can be seen as one who may be dull or directionless. These are broad sweeping generalizations, yet most people have *some* associations attached to particular decorating styles. When you break down the cognitive process of why we are drawn to certain styles or themes to surround ourselves with, it basically comes down to what makes us feel comfortable, and in turn that reflects our attitudes and behaviors. When looking at a stranger's choice of furnishing and fixtures, it is natural to come to certain conclusions about them. These subjective impressions often guide us to subconscious conclusions. It doesn't take much of a cerebral stretch to see the parallels in decorating choices to personality predilections.

When I teach an interior design course, I like to give students a handout that has a list of decorating styles (shabby chic, ethnic, retro, rustic, etc.) on one column and another column with a mix of pro and con personality traits (reliable, rigid, determined, pretentious, etc.). I ask my students, who range from established interior designers to curious do-it-yourselfers, to describe the best and worst personality traits associated with particular interior decorating styles. This exercise always causes passionate debates that the class enjoys. The "answers," as we can mostly agree on, can be subjective. (However, when I average a hundred surveys, nearly 95 percent agree on the following negative traits: Traditional style decorators are categorized as "predictable," and those who favor baroque are looked upon as "pretentious." Those who have "no design style" are considered "dull.") So there are some general stereotypes that hold up when drawing assumptions, which are interesting, but I encourage my students to examine this more fully. As one student told me, "My brother is twenty-five and his entire apartment is all formal and baroque. And he is not stuffy or pretentious whatsoever." To me, the combination of a young, single guy with a casual, low-key demeanor, as she described, seemed at odds in such a proper and ornate setting. After some discussion, it turns out this is the style they grew up in. In starting out on his own, it was all he knew in trying to create a sense of a "grown up" home for himself that he hoped to flip soon. I'm betting that in time, he will eventually find his own style—maybe a pared-down or modern baroque, or maybe a completely different style—as he finds his own voice.

This brings us to evaluating your own style and determining if your style truly supports who you are and where you'd like to be. If you feel like you cannot fairly evaluate your own interior decorating style, try asking trusted friends and visitors how they would describe the style of your décor. An additional way is to look in your own closet to determine your clothing style and see if your interior decorating choices clash or complement your clothing style and vice versa. If a significant disparity is revealed, you may want to reevaluate your style choices and ask yourself if you really feel comfortable in your immediate environment (clothes) and your spatial environment (home). My mother's shell motif is just as predominate in her wardrobe as her living space. It works for her.

A good friend I know with a high-powered job in the fashion retail industry values her moments to unwind and de-stress. She has closets of truly extraordinary designer clothes, yet also great amounts of sweat pants and casual attire. Her apartment is a reflection of high-quality furnishings mixed with thrifty and casual ones. She is comfortable in her own skin, and that's reflected in both her clothes and her apartment. I know another gal who only dresses in casual, loose, baggy clothing, yet her home has not one comfortable and relaxed place to plunge into. Her only couch is a hard-backed, petite Queen Anne style two-seater. There's a disconnect there. It's a thought-provoking exercise to examine both your wardrobe and décor to see if both expressions of your style are complementary and accommodating of who you are. Once you have determined it, ask yourself if you are satisfied with your surroundings and if you are ready to enhance what you currently have or if you are ready for a change.

MY STORY: STYLE VERSUS LIFESTYLE INSIDE MY HOME

My wardrobe preference can be broken down pretty simply: worn jeans and a cashmere sweater in winter and tons of casual white linen dresses in summer. I like well-made shoes and bags. When I have to kick it up a notch for classes, clients, or events, I enjoy dressing up, but I'm most comfortable being casual. I could easily stay in on a winter day just writing, wearing sweatpants, and making stew in the slow cooker, and it makes me extremely happy. On occasion, I even walk the dog and take my daughter to the bus in the early morning wearing the same clothes I slept

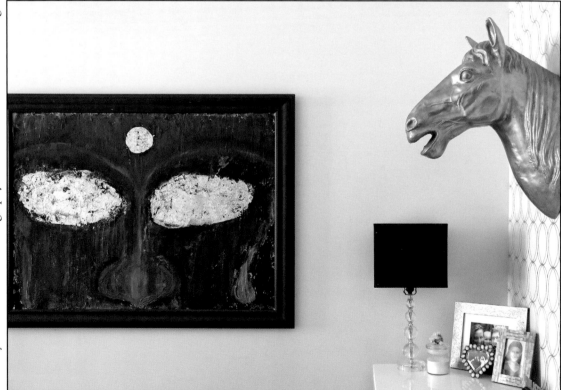

Courtesy of Susan Fisher Photography/Architecture, Interiors & Design.

in, because at that hour I'm not the priority, and I have no self-consciousness about that.

I love simple objects of beauty, and I tend to bring them in with accessories—pocketbooks, shoes, scarves, and Satya jewelry. When I think of the décor of my own home, it's pretty similar in the sense that there's comfortable pieces mixed with some special items here and there and some dashes of luxury. Fabrics, drapes, and throw rugs are all natural fibers, but there are (I'm going to refrain from using the most overused design phrase in history: "pops of color") bits of bright hues, shiny metallics, and meaningful artwork.

I have lighting fixtures, desks, a chair, and other items in my home that I procured from Craigslist.

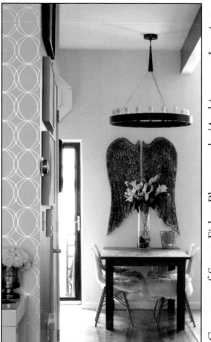

Courtesy of Susan Fisher Photography/Architecture, Interiors & Design

I find it to be a great resource. I tell people all the time: First, do an online search for the items you want, and then go to Craigslist.org in your area and see if it's available there. Why pay full price for the exact item that you want when you may find it for much less than that? There are also Facebook marketplaces in your area that buy and sell items. You have to be careful when dealing with and meeting up with strangers, and there are online scams that can arise; just be smart in your searches and always bring along someone else when you go to look at the item for sale. I found my reclaimed teak farm table because a woman bought one that turned out to be too small for her needs. She told me that it sat "like a postage stamp in the middle of my dining room" for a week while she ordered the next size up. When that was about to arrive, she needed to get this one out immediately, and I was able to score it for a third of the price. Deals like this can happen all the time. eBay and garage sales are other great bets. I always make sure I clean and sage whatever items I bring in. If I ever get a feeling I don't like about the person, I won't buy it. Also, call it superstitious, but if someone is selling something because of a negative situation like a nasty divorce or bankruptcy, I'm not eager to buy it. Of course they could always lie or not inform me of the situation, but that's where sage comes in handy.

In contrast, I have other pieces that are brand-new, investments, or custom-made. A lot of the artwork is from friends or painted by me. My daughter has made lots of paintings and sculpture pieces, which I love to display. One of my most treasured collections comes from my mom, Barbara Benko, who is a phenomenal, award-winning portrait painter. She found her calling in her retirement and can realistically paint anyone flawlessly from a photograph. There are lots of handmade pieces such as our large mirror that my husband wrapped using discarded tin that he found at the curb; a friend welded an iron coffee table that we topped with Carrara marble; and my daughter's room has a shelf my husband made from turquoise reclaimed lumber.

My bedroom wallpaper is grass cloth backed with shiny, recycled Mylar. I describe it as what I aim to be on a good day—natural, with a little bit of glamour. As my own needs and tastes have changed, as well as my husband's and daughter's, our home has reflected that. When my daughter Luchia grew out of her pink and brown bedroom with a brass

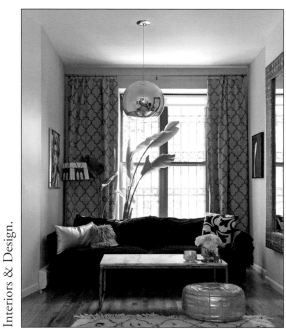

bed and wanted a modern beach-themed room, my husband and I did it ourselves.

On a daily basis, a candle is lit with intention or incense is burned to ground the atmosphere. My one indulgence is fresh flowers. Arranging them myself is therapeutic, and nearly every room has some of these earthly splendors. There might also be creative messes here and there that foster my daughter's inventiveness or show some poor time management on my part, but at the end of the day, a clean sweep puts most stuff back in its place so it doesn't snowball into a huge mess.

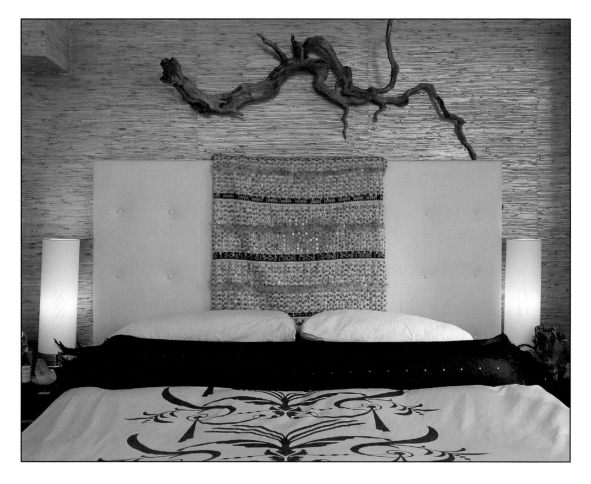

Much like my wardrobe, my gathered sense of décor that I like reflects the needs and tastes of my varied lifestyle. This creates an atmosphere that feels centered and balanced for me. I'd define my current décor style as eclectic/modern/Moroccan/rustic. But a soulful and balanced home can certainly be all one style. It's the *gathering and meaning behind it all*, combined with the predominant energy of what occurs there, that helps usher in a feeling of warmth, personalization, and soul.

CASE STUDY: REGINA WEISCHEIT

Regina Weisheit is as warm and welcoming as her home. "I like going into junk shops, tag sales, and flea markets," she says. She has a keen eye for design and purchased items

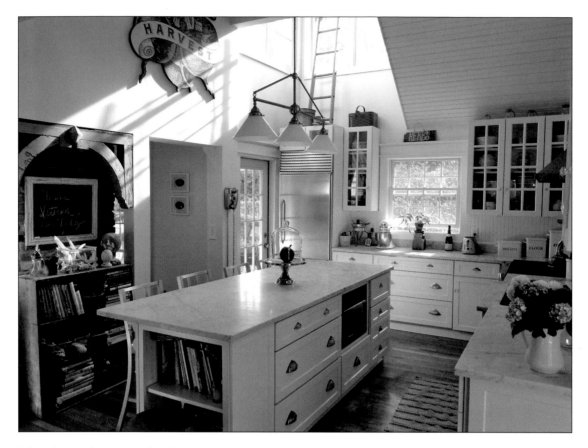

like the architectural salvage elements seen here above the chalkboard, the bookcase, the large HARVEST sign, and the ladder on top of the refrigerator without even knowing where they would fit. "I buy things that I like and they eventually find a place." Her two tips for creating a home with soul are, first, "Fill it only with objects that you absolutely love . . . *and* that you will absolutely use," and her second tip is my favorite: "Don't nickel-and-dime yourself when it comes to the one big, statement piece that you love. Most people hesitate to do this and end up buying lots of other little, cheaper stuff they don't want that end up costing the same or more in the end." After years of teaching friends how to pull together a room by thoughtfully gathering, mixing styles, and repurposing, her services as a design coach/shopper are in high demand because she helps you find your voice and lets it shine in your home.

In Regina and her husband John's lake house, featured on pages 151–153, the "soul" of the home comes from the amalgamation of John's handiwork and her

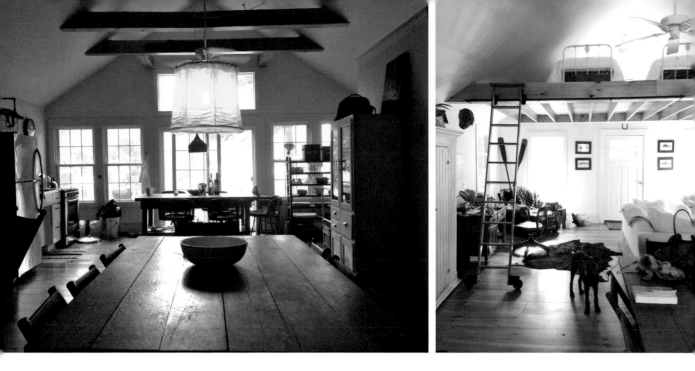

discerning eye for "rustic/camp/industrial/ lake house" décor with meaning. John completely gutted and then raised the ceilings from low to cathedral by taking out a crawl space.

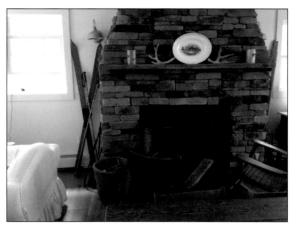

He installed new windows, wide-planked floorboards, and a hefty rein-forcement beam to create a clever sleeping loft. The first floor was completely reconfigured, and one bedroom was made into two. A couple of friends along the way helped out, but John did nearly all of the work by himself, often staying at the home in the bitter cold for five days at a time, working day and night with just a bed, table, and toaster oven.

I was shocked to learn that John didn't even know how to do most of this type of construction work beforehand, but he would watch YouTube videos and tutorials online to tackle these projects. He even added the wood-burning stone fireplace above.

Regina's scores run the gamut from tag sales, flea markets, thrift shops, Craigslist, and antique shops, and are effortlessly gathered with an uncontrived simplicity that are fitting for a rustic lake house.

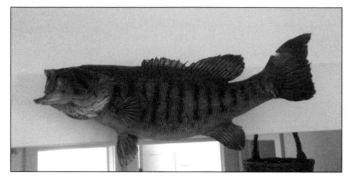

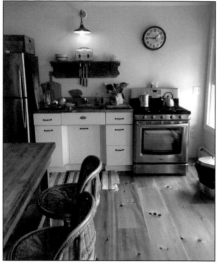

It's a home where every detail comes together—from the camp-like silverware to the Civil War iron twin beds to the mounted fish that John and Regina saved and brought back to life from a shop they said was filled with "complete trash."

The Tracy sink pictured above was a $100 treasure from the old Levitt homes; John painted the cabinet and added knobs. Above the sink shines a light fixture that John found at his mother's house and wired and mounted according to Regina's vision.

"Custom shades can be expensive, so right now I'm just using tea towels on the windows!" Even her clever fold is creative and does the job.

"I like displaying odd things . . . elements of nature . . . things I find beautiful. This beehive is beautiful to me."

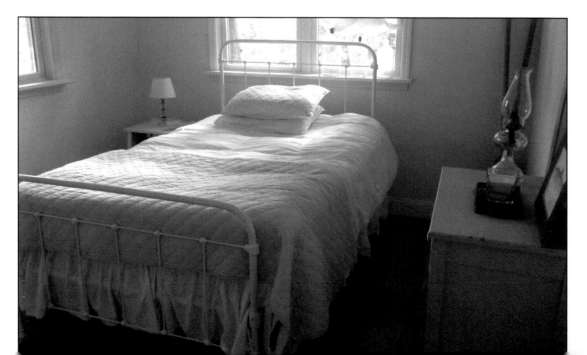

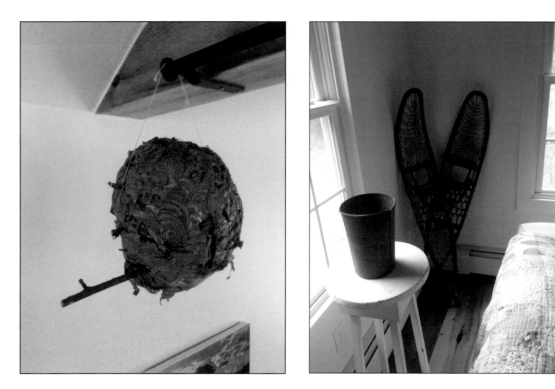

Is Your Home Environment the Best It Can Be?
Ask Yourself These Three Questions:

1. When was the last time you updated your décor?

If it has been more than five years ago, consider making updates, even on a small level. Change displayed items, collectibles, or artwork to reflect a fresh perspective, a new beginning in your life, or to open yourself to a phase that you hope to happen. If you have experienced a major life change, such as death, divorce, or a move, it is best to get a new mattress and try different paint colors as soon as possible.

2. Does my home reflect not only my current needs, but where I would like to be in the future?

A great way to usher in new life changes is to set up your home to accommodate them. A hobby or exercise space can be inspiring and motivating to recent empty nesters that now have an extra room. A new guest room that was once an underused office can be solace to a lonely occupant. Ask yourself what you feel you are lacking in your life. No matter what the answer is (creativity, visitors, health, organization, spirituality), once you create and designate the space with focused intention, you are opening the flow of energy to what is needed.

3. When I enter my home, do I feel happy, relaxed, and at peace?

For some people, when they walk through the door, it's not quite Home Sweet Home. The reasons can vary. The most common ones I've heard: a daunting list of unfinished home projects; a great deal of disorganization; uninspiring, lifeless décor; or unpleasant memories. Each one of these issues can eventually be transformed. Tackling the clutter is the first step (chapter 2) to diminishing chaos and can greatly reduce stress. We all have running to-do lists. But by systematically approaching each chore, from small to large, and taking time to acknowledge the sense of accomplishment after each task completion, unfinished business will not feel so daunting. After organizing your space, clear the psychic residue of your home with a sage clearing. This allows the predecessor energy to be released and opens the energetic pathways for clean, clear, and fresh energy to enter. Once organization has been put in place and the energies of the space have been consecrated, the fun part of decorating with intention and meaning can begin.

HOLISTIC HOME DECORATING GUIDELINES

Avoid decorating with plastic. That means everything from vertical vinyl blinds to plastic flowers. Vertical blinds are like knives in Feng Shui that create harsh angles of chi. Plastics are made from noxious chemicals and can off-gas, plus they have an inorganic, lifeless essence, which greatly diminishes the energy in your home and in yourself.

Bring in nature. Try to use fresh flowers when possible or at least a plant in every room. An element of nature can also be a massive crystal, or a collection of shells, driftwood, or branches in a vase. A client had a large cylindrical glass vase filled with dozens of layers of sand that varied in color and texture. It was not only visually beautiful, but each layer told a story of her coastal travels around the world. Your nature gatherings can even be seasonal—a bowl of pinecones in winter can be changed out for a bowl of water and flower petals in spring. When you honor nature inside your home, you are tapping into a restorative energy, honoring your interconnectedness on this planet, and creating a bit of balance in our mostly man-made home environments.

Take your time. When you move into a new home, don't feel you need to have it completely decorated right away. It can take a while to figure it all out, from the sunlight patterns for paint selections to realizing how each room is truly being utilized. Decorating your home should be a journey in treasure collecting; otherwise, it can end up looking like a standard hotel room or a dull, discount furniture commercial.

Make mistakes. Sometimes the errors we make in decorating end up either teaching us a lesson (measure twice, cut once!) or giving us a surprise gift (that couch table didn't fit in the living room but it's fantastic in the entryway!). Allow yourself the freedom to fall. It's very common for blunders to turn to beauties. When I used a high-gloss enamel paint with my oversized stencil on the inside of my closet door, I was dismayed when I took off the stencil and saw how the white paint imperfectly bled onto the cinnabar background. I sat with it for a couple days as I contemplated the resolution, but then realized I absolutely loved the look of it. I purposely tried to replicate that look as I continued the stencil pattern.

Refresh every few years. Stuck in an era? Be sure to update your decorating so you are not living in the past. If you have the same hairstyle from high school and you're now in your forties, chances are your décor needs a refresher too. It's great to decorate with styles inspired by particular eras, but be sure to do a décor evaluation every few years so your home will grow and evolve—just like you are. A home that has not had a decorating update in decades produces a stale energy, which fosters a rigid mindset. If you are stuck in the past with your décor, your thinking will be too.

Get inspired. Inspiration can come from anywhere. Television decorating shows, vacations, hotels, restaurants, nature, Internet searches, home tours, home furnishing catalogs, design magazines, and books. Just look around you. Notice what draws you, what repels you, and build from there. Take frequent pictures with your phone to capture any images you love. Create an inspiration folder with photos, tear sheets, printouts, swatches, or catalogues; use Pinterest or Instagram to collect looks you love. Next, look through what you've gathered and try to see if there is a theme or a thread of connection. Take that idea and go from there.

Find meaning. Strive to surround yourself with objects, accessories, collectibles, and artwork that hold an enjoyable significance to you. Don't look to buy art just because of how it matches your couch or because you feel it was a good investment. If you are buying art just for investment's sake, don't bother unless you're a dealer. The precious treasures you choose for your surroundings should inspire a strong and positive visceral reaction. Some of the most common regret-filled descriptions I hear involve paying too much or keeping an unwanted item because it was a gift. If you want to be happy, make the choice to surround yourself with the things that make you feel that way.

Edit. Yes, you should surround yourself with items you love, but don't go overboard. "It started off because I liked owls when I was a kid. [Then] practically every gift from friends and family was owl related. I've become an unintentional hoarder of owls. It's out of control." Suzy felt overwhelmed easily. The hundred-plus owls in her home were not helping. Once she whittled her collection down to nine, she felt freer, lighter, and ready for a fresh start. Unlike most classic hoarders, Suzy was ready to let go and make a change, which is the hardest part. If you have an excessive amount of collectibles, reduce them down and display them in one spot, not all over the house. This creates a dramatic and purposeful impact without feeling cluttered.

Don't be afraid of open spaces. A room filled with too much furniture leads to a cluttered mind. Allow the chi to flow and not be jammed up in a furniture or knickknack jumble. Just when you think you have the right amount, go in and edit again.

IT IS YOUR HOUSE. YOU ARE IN CHARGE.

When I am doing a consultation on a home that has been decorated by an interior designer and not by the occupants, it becomes an additional layer to unveil to get to the core issues. Good interior decorators can encourage a client to go to design boundaries they never imagined, so for clients who are creatively timid, insecure about their own design decisions, or use the excuse that they "are too busy" to put effort into their own surroundings, then perhaps this kind of guidance can be helpful. However, even with the best-intentioned and well-respected designers, they are still creating an environment that says, "This is how I see you." Even when the designer gathers "choices" for their client to pick from, it is still the designer's wheelhouse that it is coming from. The goal is find an interior designer that really listens, knows you well and truly respects your input. If you're in the market, there are many talented ones out there, you just have to spend time to find the one that is right for you.

Often issues will surface surrounding the decorating process for the occupants, such as feeling taken advantage of, difficulty speaking up, losing one's sense of self, or a general feeling of conflict. These feelings may or may not be directed toward your interior decorator at the time but are very common emotions to surface when someone else is creating and executing the vision for your personal space. Surely most interactions with professional decorators go smoothly, but if there is even a shred of their ego involved, issues involving a loss of voice or identity and increased discord will be launched to the surface for the occupants. If you must use one, try to find a decorator that fits your personality, meets your budget, and has flexibility with final design decisions. Remember, you are paying the interior designer to realize your vision in your own home, not to create his or her *own* vision.

Over time, living in a beautiful place that is filled with someone else's ideas can weaken your individual chi and sense of purpose. Although it may look great, the decorator's thumbprint will be a ubiquitous reminder, manifesting subtle energetic ramifications that are not conducive to a home that supports the individuality, the interests, and the sense of harmony of you and those who live there.

If your space was professionally decorated, it does not mean that you are surely headed for an identity crisis; it just means that you might want to reflect on the root of the choices that were made as well as your own honest feelings surrounding them. Part of having the inexplicable feeling of "soul" in your home is that your home is a personalized creation from *you*.

ELLEN: IT'S CURTAINS FOR HER DOMINANT DESIGNER

Ellen called me for a consultation because she wanted to find a meaningful relationship. It's more the norm in my consultations to address the core issues as they come up because that's the only way a real change is going to happen. Here, I had to try to get to get to the emotional underpinnings of Ellen's self-worth and then draw the clear connections to her environment before I could even start making suggestions to create a balanced and welcoming atmosphere for a relationship. During the consultation, she said she was full of regret for hiring an interior designer that she clashed with. She pointed to lavish silk curtains and cried, "She even lined the back of the curtains with silk. I spent way too much money and ended up hating it all." Although this Fifth Avenue apartment in Manhattan looked lovely and could be featured in a magazine, Ellen was miserable. She mentioned that she preferred dating dominant-minded men, and during the consultation she also referred to her interior designer many times as "dominant." Once we started talking and she relayed stories of past boyfriends, it seemed the "dominant men" she dated were more of a bully than just a powerful or confident man with a take-charge attitude.

Her feelings of being taken advantage of by her overly persuasive interior designer mirrored her unhappy patterns of consistently choosing overly dominant men. Both made her feel compliant and passive. In the end, both made her unhappy and very resentful. The domineering designer's choices were ensconcing Ellen in a home that was not allowing her own voice to be heard. Everywhere Ellen looked were constant reminders of her own passivism, which fueled a silent rage. This wasn't an easy consultation. Ellen was not pleased with me when I pointed out this pattern and drew the connections to her space. I get it. I scratched the surface and it hurt. Ellen only wanted to hear recommendations to help bring in a relationship. However, in order to invite a balanced relationship into her life, she needed to deal with the issues that propelled her to attract domineering energy and break that pattern. I did not push Ellen. What she needed was to take this to a therapist to delve deeper into her own issues of self-worth and her inability to speak up. I did let her know that reclaiming her voice would get easier with the removal of any unwanted design elements. I told Ellen that although hiring an interior decorator was a huge expense, I suggested she allow herself time to reflect on removing what represented the most resentment to her. In turn, the emotional benefits would be priceless.

The curtains were the most energetically loaded remnant that needed to go. As Ellen opened the heavy curtains, the light came streaming in, and I told her that in Feng Shui windows represent the eyes and our own clarity. The symbolic gesture of removing these heavy window coverings that represented her loss of self could be an empowering insight for her. I told her, "Let your own uniqueness shine through.

Let your voice speak up and fill this space now." I encouraged her to make reflective choices by asking, "Do I love it? Does it represent me, my interests, and the person I'd like to be?" The rest would hopefully sort itself out. The more Ellen would strengthen her environment, the more her inner environment of self would be fortified. It's not about living in a space that is a magazine showplace. It's about creating a home that reinforces and supports you in all ways possible.

> ### The Most Common Thing I See in Every Home: Fear
> Fear manifests the most transparently in your space. It comes to the surface quickly and in varied ways, such as the positioning of your mirrors or the clutter on your shelves. When you know what to look for, the manifestations of fear are easy to identify, and removing them leaves you and your home ready for your soul to shine. (Refer to pages 31–32 to evaluate the table on types of fears.)

JANE: INADEQUATE BY DESIGN

Jane's experience with her interior designer, Julia, was not problematic during the process. "We got along fine, she's great! I work twelve-hours days and would not call myself the least bit creative. At first I liked my home in the same way you'd walk into a friend's well-decorated home and admire it. But now that several months have passed, I find that I'm just reminded of how inadequate I am. Could I have done a better job? I don't think so. But at this point, I don't like living here. People ask me about my antique car horn collection, and I don't know what to tell them except Julia thought it was quirky! It feels like I had to have someone else create my own quirky persona, and it makes me feel less than. I don't even care about antique horns or the color green, but Julia said green reminded her of me, and now my entire living room—rug to ceiling—is green." Jane had just recently broken up with her boyfriend, yet seemed to be doing fine with that dissolution since she kept lightheartedly referring to him as "Mr. All Wrong."

Months after the consultation, Jane unexpectedly had to move to Miami. She sold her home furnished with everything in it. (I'm assuming the car horn collection too!) Her new home has no leftovers of her old place, and she emailed me an update: "Slowly decorating my new condo. Loving it. I may be breaking all design rules but it is ME and I don't feel like I am trying to be someone I am not. Dating someone new. Happiest I've been in a long time." Another positive side to this is that Jane's experience with her interior designer had eventually inspired her to personally create the home that she always wanted—but thought she didn't know how to create. Perhaps Jane needed the catalyst of living in an environment that was not her own, only to come to the realization of her own potential. Jane said it best: "Just like my love life, sometimes we gotta experience what we don't want in order to ultimately get to know what we do." Makes sense to me.

MOVING INTO AN ALREADY FURNISHED HOME

Furnished sublets or already-purchased fully furnished homes have a longer adjustment period of settling in, and the home will not be energetically in tandem with your personal goals and desires—until adjustments are made. If you are already living in an environment like this, try to work on ways to put your thumbprint in the home. If you are staying in this environment temporarily, make small but significant adjustments every day to make it your own. Bring in flowers; arrange them with care, and place them in a spot you see the most. Move around the furniture to create a new arrangement that suits you, and bring in accessories and photographs to personalize the space.

DO IT YOURSELF

Mammoth household tasks like removing asbestos, plumbing, or wiring electricity—hire a professional. When it comes to filling your house with the things you love—you can do it yourself. Times are changing. Vendors that once only sold to the trade are now opening to the public. More and more people are gaining the confidence to decorate their homes themselves. Design blogs like Apartment Therapy and Design*Sponge offer endless design concepts that are unique, creative, and inspiring. Some furniture stores are bridging gaps by offering on-staff interior designers to advise in the general process of doing it all on your own. A new trend now with interior designers is a service that offers a one-time consultation to help get you on track. Living in an environment that you created—mistakes and all—is always more empowering than one you did not.

COLOR

Color has a certain vibrational tone that chi picks up and redistributes back out into the environment. Even though everyone's perception of color is subjective, our biological vision is universal. Light reflected off different surfaces passes through the cornea and then stimulates the optical nerve system. Colors have varying wavelengths: Red, orange, and yellow have long wavelengths that stimulate and energize. Green is neutral. Blues and purples have short wavelengths that relax and calm us.

In addition to the science, there are definite widespread psychological associations with color that are commonly held. Red conjures up images of authority (a red "power" tie, walking the red carpet). It is a strong Yang color that is considered lucky in Feng Shui. It expels bad chi and can act as a stimulator. Too much and it breeds an aggressive environment. Orange is an uplifting, stimulating color that promotes happiness. Yellow or gold symbolizes power, and stimulates health, patience, and wisdom.

Green can represent growth and new beginnings (recycling and reusing are synonyms for being "green") as well as healing and freshness. Blues with green undertones, like turquoise, represent youth and new beginnings, and inspire confidence. Deeper blues like sapphire and indigo infuse wisdom and introspection; however, in ancient Chinese culture, this shade is a secondary mourning color. Purple inspires spirituality, adventure, power, and prosperity. Black is a contemplative color that encourages reflection and mystery. White cultivates clarity, precision, and communication. Gray invites helpfulness and represents a harmonious union of black and white. Brown offers stability and security. Pink represents love, romance, and partnership.

DECORATING WITH THE ELEMENTS

In chapter 3, the Five Elements, their properties, and how they are symbolized and represented were discussed. Below are decorating examples of how each element can be used in its design form, and the pros and cons when they are out of balance.

Fire

The color red, triangular shapes, and actual fire represent the element Fire. By painting with fiery tones, using candles, adding red fabrics or accessories, you can ignite passions and spark motivation. If used too much, it can promote aggression and irritability. Too little in an environment and it feels cold and lacks purpose.

Wood

In addition to real wood furniture and accessories, the Wood element is found in rich greens, plants, flowers, wicker, and tall, upright shapes. An overabundance of wood creates an energy of stubbornness and feeling overwhelmed. The Wood element is great for children's rooms, since it works in tandem with their growing energy. A deficiency of wood in your home can stagnate growth and creativity.

Water

Water is a powerful element to add to your environment in its exact element form by using a clean water feature, such as a water fountain, a fish tank, or even a simple bowl of water with some floating petals. Moving water in a fountain enhances spirituality, wealth, and relaxation. A water fountain also humidifies the air and releases negative ions, which clean the air and make breathing easier. Water helps elucidate your thinking, but too much can make you feel spacey and unfocused. Artwork that depicts water can work to symbolize this element, but choose the image carefully for the right room. Do you want the rousing force of crashing waves or a serene beach landscape that soothes?

Asymmetrical shapes and the color black symbolize water. A curving coffee table or a black couch are examples of bringing in the water element. A lack of water present can lead to tension and sarcasm in that environment.

Metal

Metal enhances communication and mental focus and reduces confusion and procrastination. Bring it into your home in areas where mental clarity is preferred, such as the kitchen and home office. This element is found in all metal objects—brass, gold, silver, nickel, copper, steel, and in metal furniture. The metal element is symbolized by the color white and dome shapes. A home lacking in white and metal elements will promote indecisive and confused energy. An excess of metal creates self-righteousness and stubbornness.

Earth

The power of Earth supports physical strength, practicality, and stability. Too much Earth and the home can feel heavy and serious; not enough and the home will feel unstable and chaotic. Earth is represented in the color yellow and earthen elements like adobe, tile, ceramic, and brick.

MIRRORS

Mirrors are one of the most important Feng Shui adjustments that you can use. Avoid unclear mirrors with a heavy antique-like patina. Mirrors help redirect the flow of chi, open up the space of a room, and create expansiveness for the particular gua that they are

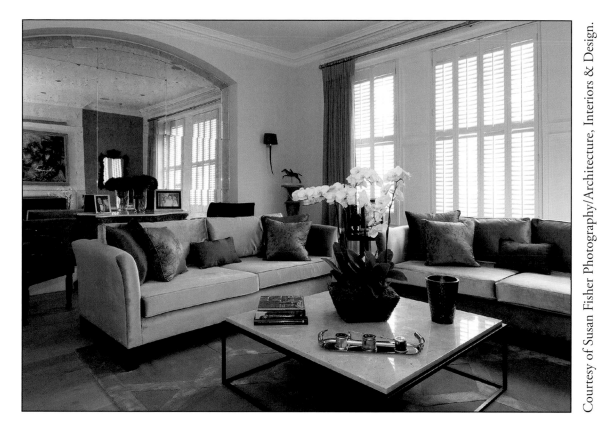

Courtesy of Susan Fisher Photography/Architecture, Interiors & Design.

placed in. Make sure the mirrors are not hung too high (occupants will feel uncomfortable, feel low self-esteem, or feel as if they can never measure up) or too low (headaches will be prevalent). Always be mindful of what you are reflecting—is it the television or a pile of bills? Not a good idea. That image will be doubled. Rethink placement.

Try to position or install mirrors so you are reflecting more natural light or a nice view from outside.

STRUCTURAL ELEMENTS: STAIRS, WINDOWS, AND DOORS

Spiral staircases are not energetically beneficial because of their corkscrew-like formation, which dramatically accelerates energy up and down. Staircases without riser backs allow the chi to escape in between each step and create an unstable home environment. Ideally, stairs should be broad, well lit, and not pointing toward your front door or up to your bathroom. If the stairs are the first thing that you see when you enter your home, anchor the chi at the top of the stairs with rocks, statues, or potted plants.

Windows represent the eyes. Too big and the chi will be rushing in too quickly. If the windows are too small, seeing the "bigger picture" in life will be a challenge. It is important that the glass always be clear and clean. If you are at a crossroads about a decision, a great Feng Shui exercise is to clean the window as you reflect on an answer.

Your front door is the mouth of chi. It must be clearly marked and lit, with nothing obstructing it. If the front gets stuck easily, your life challenges will increase in frustration. Good colors are red, black, and green. Interior doors should not hit other doors when opening. This is called "conflicting doors" and leads to domestic arguments. To adjust for conflicting doors, try installing pocket doors or a sliding door with a rolling apparatus on the top and bottom.

KIDS AND DECORATING

If you have young children, you can still have a put-together home without it looking like a daycare. My rule of thumb: the more valuable/expensive/risky the item, the higher it should be located in the room. A tall dresser or shelf is the perfect place to showcase an invaluable collection of treasures, fragile items, or a burning candle. When you have kids, indulge in artwork on the walls or statement ceiling light fixtures, but buy less precious items for the lower half of the room—like rugs, floor pillows, ottomans, storage baskets,

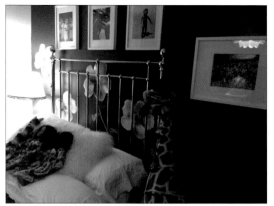

certain low seating, and so forth. If your couch covers and throw rugs can be thrown in the wash, your life will be much, much easier!

Kids grow fast, and their spaces should be updated accordingly—approximately every two to three years. A fresh room that reflects their changing tastes and contains furniture that is appropriate for their age (or the age they soon will be) will easily embrace their next growth cycle. Everything in the room should be thoroughly organized with a designated place for every item. Symbolism should be calming (avoid transportation motifs); jarring primary colors should be avoided. Choose more of the Wood and Earth elements, because they support growth while creating security.

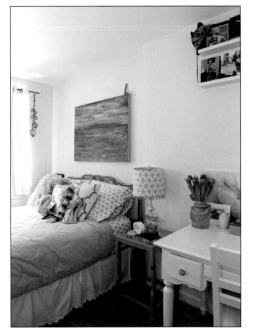

Courtesy of Susan Fisher Photography/Architecture, Interiors & Design

If children are going through a difficult time, such as a divorce, a move, or an illness, it is essential that their room feel solid and stable. This means their bed or crib should be in a commanding position with nothing underneath it. Bunk beds are fine for kids' rooms, but be sure to add a small round mirror directly above both of the heads of the children (from the perspective of lying with their head on the pillow, looking up toward the ceiling). This Feng Shui adjustment helps redirect the oppressive energy that both sleepers could feel.

Try to get your children involved in taking responsibility in their own room through routines and hands-on action. When kids make their bed every morning, it sets the tone for a prepared day and instills personal pride in their space. Start by doing it with them; have fun and use it as an opportunity to connect about the day. Encourage them to put their things away at the end of the day. Not only will that rein in larger messes, but it also creates a sense of stability through routine and purpose. These routines can become the foundation for teaching your child about management, organization, and strategy.

ELECTROMAGNETIC FIELDS

Electromagnetic fields (EMFs) are getting a great deal of attention lately. Studies suggest that being barraged with EMFs can have potentially harmful side effects.

EMFs are created by electric power charges; therefore, they are found all around you, radiating from computers, microwaves, cell phones, transformers, electrical appliances, TVs, and fluorescent lighting. There are two types of fields—electric fields that result from the strength (voltage) of the charge, and magnetic fields, which result from the motion (amperage) of the charge.

Data strongly suggest that when we are constantly being bombarded by a myriad of man-made electromagnetic energy, biological dangers can occur. These EMFs induce internal currents, which are then spatially averaged over the entire body, specifically affecting the brain and growing tissue. Keep in mind that we are all electrical beings. Our bodies are made up of millions of fine-tuned electrical circuits, and every time our heart beats or we move a muscle, there are electrical neuronal discharges. Brain waves, heartbeats, cell division, bone growth, and all sensory information that move through our body are electrical. EMFs are believed to interfere with that biochemistry.

Debates currently continue with verve as far as how harmful the biological effects are, but some research has found that certain blood and brain cancers are related to EMF exposure as well as headaches, chronic fatigue, visual disturbances, inability to concentrate, malaise, eyestrain, infertility, mild panic, and fetal abnormalities. Pregnant women and children should be particularly mindful about EMF exposure because their cells are growing at a much faster rate.

The bottom line is this: move electrical appliances and devices at least thirty inches from your head—especially where you spend most of your time, like your bed. There are ceramic converters or diodes available that diffuse the chaotic wavelengths from EMF offenders and have been found to assuage negative environments tremendously.

ECO-CONSCIOUS CHOICES IN FURNITURE, LIGHTING, FABRICS, AND MORE

The chemicals that make plastic pliant and flame-resistant are considered the most toxic on the planet. The omnipresent role of plastic in our lives is causing significant disruptions in thyroid and endocrine functions. Organic materials, natural fabrics, and natural lighting are imbued with healthy chi; therefore, choosing them over synthetic products and fluorescent lighting can enhance and strengthen your chi. When you decrease the toxicities in your environment, you are decreasing the toxicities within yourself, not just physically but spiritually and emotionally. It's never too late to detox your décor and make healthier choices.

Wood Furniture

Avoid particleboard or pressed wood, as it may contain formaldehyde. Choose sustainably harvested woods, and look for items that bear the FSC (Forest Stewardship Council) certification. There are both pros and cons to using the old-growth, large-diameter trees and rare hardwoods. The harder woods last longer and won't need to be replaced like the quick-growing and much softer bamboo. However, they must be responsibly managed by not overharvesting, or the trees must have fallen naturally. There are some unique engineered boarding options that outperform many other woods in strength, shrinking, and warping, such as Kirei, which is constructed from leftover sorghum stalks and contains no formaldehyde.

Lighting

Compact fluorescent bulbs—although energy-efficient and cost-effective—give off larger amounts of electromagnetic fields and also contain mercury. If broken, you have created a hazardous waste situation inside your home that initially causes dizziness and nausea and then eventually can damage your nervous system. If this occurs, toxicology experts recommend getting out of the house for at least twenty minutes. When you return, use gloves to sweep the pieces into a bag and then dispose of at a hazardous waste collection site. Fluorescent bulbs also subtly flicker, which can set off migraines and are problematic for epileptics.

This type of lighting is often chosen for stores and offices because it is cheap. At the very least, most people who are in tune with their bodies can feel the negative effects of massive fluorescent lighting overhead for a length of time. Remember that the light that radiates on us is just as important as the quality of air that we breathe. Full spectrum lightbulbs mimic natural wavelength patterns of sunlight most accurately. A reasonable solution may be to have compact fluorescent bulbs in places where you do not spend a great deal of time sitting, such as exterior light fixtures, closets, and the garage and basement.

Fabrics and Textures

Try to select organic, natural fiber textiles, such as organic cotton, jute, silk, wool, bamboo, linen, or hemp. Make sure it does not have a fire-retardant or stain-resistant treatment, which can disrupt endocrine function. For pillows and cushion inserts, avoid polyurethane foam because of its petroleum base and chemical outgases, and instead choose non-GMO soy or corn-based fiber fill or organic cotton stuffing.

Texture is discovered through touch: rough, smooth, coarse, velvety, and silky are examples. Texture is a necessary layer in the design process that can offer visual interest, depth, and surprise. Scan each room of your home and notice what textures are missing and which are in abundance, and try to bring in variety. Bumpy grass cloth walls, a knobby pillow, silky curtains, a fluffy sheepskin rug, smooth floors, and a rough metal sculpture are examples of textures in a living room filled with varying organic textures. Mix it up so that you have varying dimensions of textures present.

Floor and Walls

Opt for sustainable wood floors, stone or ceramic when possible. Choose mats or area rugs that can easily be shaken out and washed. Avoid wall-to-wall synthetic carpeting, which may contain carcinogens, chemicals, and fire retardants. Jute, wool, hemp, raffia, sea grass, abaca, silk, cork, or sisal are beautiful and healthy alternatives to synthetic carpets, and actually several of these options (raffia, sea grass, silk, cork) can be used on your walls too. Wallpaper has undergone a huge transformation from the vinyl of decades past and comes in vibrant colors and dynamic patterns.

KEEPING IT CLEAN AND CLEAR

Our shoes track in an estimated 85 percent of the dirt in our homes. Remove them before entering, and you are also cutting down on 60 percent of lead dust levels in your home, according to the Environmental Protection Agency. Making your own "green" cleaning supplies is easy and cheap. Use hydrogen peroxide instead of chlorine bleach to disinfect. Use one part white vinegar to two parts water as an all-purpose household cleaner. Use a teaspoon of lemon juice in a pint of vegetable oil for furniture polish. Always make sure that you have air circulating in your home—whether it's a window slightly open, a ceiling fan, or an air purifier; a stagnant home can feel suffocating and lifeless.

INVITING SPIRITUALITY INTO YOUR HOME

Having visual reminders of spirituality in your home, such as a garden Buddha statue, a mezuzah on your door frame, or a picture of a saint on the wall are great if you have a deep connection to these objects and they fill you with peace, comfort, or reminders of your faith when you look at them. But if that is *all* you are doing to instill spirituality in your home, you are missing out on a whole other component that can only be felt and not seen.

After reading the autobiography *Angels In My Hair* by international best-selling author Lorna Byrne, I had the opportunity to speak with her about how she can see angels as plain as you and I see each other. I asked her if our homes, like people, have guardian angels too. Byrne said no, but suggested that when we leave our homes, we should ask the angel of protection, Archangel Michael—or whatever angel we resonate with—to watch over our homes. She added that prayer enhances the invisible energies of your home, making it a place where people love being.

These invisible energies come from the predominant actions and feelings that occur inside your home. You can enhance this sacred-feeling chi by creating spiritual habits that will fill your home with a sense of sacredness. Sacred habits can be small, positive acts while visualizing your desired outcome. This can be done with simple actions from lighting a candle to cleaning the house. Every time you light a candle, hold a positive intention or make a wish and imagine it happening in vivid detail. Before you eat, gather hands around the table to share what you are happy and grateful for and focus on the good that is in your life. While cleaning your home, thank it for providing shelter and a space for memories and visualize golden, healing light ensconcing it. Create spaces in your home that encourage reflection or areas to meditate, and make sure you actually use them for that purpose. A clean and organized house has a lighter feel to it. Clutter impedes the flow of spirituality and creates a dense and heavy environment that feels anxious and ungrounded. Whatever your personal choices are for creating a sacred atmosphere, a home where spirituality prevails feels pure, light, and welcoming because it is filled with love.

The interior decoration of your home is a personal expression of who you are and who you would like to be. This journey of enhancing your intimate space can also enhance yourself along the way. With reflection and deliberate choices for your surroundings that you actively participate in, you can strengthen your voice and your goals. A home with soul is a welcoming, healthy home that holds personal meaning, inspires, and truly heralds who you are. It showcases your personality—not an idealized vision of perfection. It is a place without fear and can intrinsically help transmute the negatives that can hold you back. Don't underestimate the energetic matrix of your chosen surroundings and the importance of your role in creating a home that fearlessly expresses your soul.

CHAPTER EIGHT

Sustainable You:
Green Mind, Body, Spirit, and Space

"There is nothing like staying at home for real comfort."

—Jane Austen

A sustainable home today means more than just having a systematic recycling plan in place and the "right" lightbulbs. Today, an all-inclusive "green" environment is one that truly nourishes and supports *all aspects* of the greater whole of who you are—emotionally, physically, and spiritually.

EMOTIONAL SUSTAINABILITY

A home where mindful and sustainable actions reside embraces the senses the moment you enter it. It resonates with an elevated vibration due to its vitality and the emotions and actions of those who live there.

Add Foliage

As toxic volatile organic compounds fill your home (dry cleaning fluids, acetone, ammonia, detergents, plastics, paints, adhesives, etc.), your plants are not only scrubbing the air of these toxins, but they are doing something even a high-tech HVAC system can't. They are converting the volatile organic compounds into carbon-based materials in order to fuel photosynthesis. That means that your pretty peace lily and fluffy fern are reversing your carbon footprint while helping you breathe easier. And if that is not enough, the act of nurturing vibrant life sources in your home cultivates compassion in your environment.

The Scent of a Home

Many homes tell a story with their own unique scent, and while the aroma of certain cooking spices, hints of personal fragrance, or even beloved pets can add to that familiar scent, consider tapping into the therapeutic properties of aromatherapy as an additional green layer to instill in your home.

Discover which essential oils can help you the most. Geranium can assist in balancing hormones, lemon is an antidepressant, lavender relieves mental agitation, lemongrass enhances concentration, and peppermint revives energy. Add drops of essential oil to white vinegar/water solutions to clean just about everything in your home. Also, add essential oil drops to purified water in spray bottles instead of using conventional air fresheners. These homemade "green" cleaners and room sprays infuse the environment with restorative scents that help support you emotionally.

Try This from Jenni Hulburt

Jenni Hulburt is a health and fitness coach and wellness advocate. As the creator of the Inspire Workouts, and author of *The Dirt Detox*, she is leading the Nature Fed Wellness Movement with the goal of inspiring people to revolutionize their health through nature. Visit her for workouts, recipes, and healthy inspiration at www.jennihulburt.com.

Have you ever walked through a field of lavender or enjoyed the aroma of a freshly cut grapefruit?

You've probably experienced the power of essential oils without even realizing their impact on your well-being. Essential oils are potent aromatic extracts found in plants, used around the world as natural medicine. Essential oils embody the regenerating, oxygenating, and immune-supporting properties of plants, and there is so much more to these oils than just the aroma.

Essential oils are typically extracted via steam distillation or cold-pressing from the stem, roots, leaves, bark, or flowers of a plant. They contain hundreds of chemical compounds, making them antioxidants, antibacterial, antiviral, anti-inflammatory, antifungal, antidepressants . . . and the list goes on.

We experience many fragrances throughout the day in our environment and in our home. Many of these fragrances are synthetic versions of the plant-inspired aroma of an essential oil. For example, lavender-scented body wash or lemon-scented dish soap are made with synthetic fragrances to mimic nature. Unfortunately, synthetic aromas don't provide any health benefits, and many of them may actually be detrimental to health.

When it comes to your home, essential oils can be used in ways that support you physically, emotionally, and spiritually. The aromatic use of essential oils is simply done through inhalation and is especially good for affecting mood, air quality, and the respiratory system. Topical use of essential oils is applying them directly to the body, and is especially good to address a particular area of concern. Most high-quality oils can be used both aromatically and topically.

Essential oils are highly potent, so a little bit goes a long way. Always read the labels to be sure of their indicated use. Enjoy naturally detoxing your home—mind, body, spirit, and space with the benefits of nature! Here are some specific tips and applications for using essential oils aromatically and topically.

Aromatic

- **Direct inhalation:** Simply open the bottle and breathe, or place 1–2 drops of oil on your hands, cup the hands over the mouth and nose, and inhale.

- **Clothing and bedding:** Put 1–3 drops of an essential oil on your pillowcase, or add 10 drops to an 8-ounce spray bottle of water to spritz clothes in the dryer.
- **Room fresheners:** Add 10 drops of an essential oil to 8 ounces of water and spray as an air freshener and purifier.
- **Diffusion:** A simple way to put a fine mist of the whole essential oil into the air is by using a nebulizing diffuser. It uses room temperature air to break the oils into a micro-fine mist that is dispersed into the air. Diffusers that use an intense heat source, like a candle, are not recommended because it may alter the chemical makeup of the oil and its therapeutic qualities.
- **Multipurpose cleaner:** Mix with equal parts white vinegar and water, plus 10–15 drops essential oil in an 8-ounce spray bottle for a natural multipurpose cleaner.

Topical

- **Dish soap:** Add 10 drops to an 8-ounce bottle of liquid castile soap to clean dishes. Citrus oils, like lemon and lime, are especially good at cutting grease from pots and pans.
- **Perfume or cologne:** Apply 1–2 drops of essential oil to skin. To create a perfume, dissolve 10–15 drops of essential oil into 20 drops of alcohol and combine with 1 teaspoon distilled water. Apply as a mist to skin.
- **Bathwater:** Add 3–5 drops of oil to bathwater while the tub is filling. The skin will draw the oils from the top of the water as the water settles.
- **Bath salts:** Combine 5 drops of essential oil with ¼ cup of Epsom salts. Dissolve the salt mixture in warm bathwater before bathing.
- **Massage:** Apply 3–5 drops of an essential oil, then cover area with a hot, wet towel and a dry towel on top. The moist heat forces the oils deeper into the tissues of the body.

Uses for a Holistic Home				
Essential Oil	**Mind**	**Body**	**Spirit**	**Space**
Lemon	Creativity, focus	Detoxifying	Joy, positivity	Disinfectant for cleaning
Lavender	Anxiety	Allergies	Peace, calming	Fear of change
Eucalyptus	Concentration, focus	Respiratory support	Clear negative energy	Dispel dust mites
Cedarwood	Assertiveness	Oily skin	Relaxation	Air purification
Rosemary	Stimulating	Arthritis, pain	Confidence, opens the conscious mind	Antibacterial and antifungal
Thyme	Fatigue	Antioxidant	Uplifting, energizing	Mold
Patchouli	Anger	Skin conditions	Security	Termite repellent
Sandalwood	Antidepressant	Nervous system support	Enhance meditation	Harmonizes emotions
Ylang-ylang	Insomnia	Hormonal balance	Fear of failure, self-blame	Influences sexual energy and enhances relationships

PHYSICAL SUSTAINABILITY

The practicality of a green home on the surface seems basic, but is so vital because it affects what you see and how you dwell every day. A physically supportive eco-friendly home nourishes your body by supporting a healthy lifestyle and offers an effective approach to your day-to-day domestic needs.

Simplify Your Life

Efficiency plays a big role in sustainability. In addition to the typical ways of running an efficient household with heating, cooling, insulating, and water consumption,

Courtesy of Susan Fisher Photography/Architecture, Interiors & Design

another important aspect is in simplifying *how* you dwell every day. Surrounding yourself with only what you genuinely need and use helps diminish an endless cycle of consumption and a feeling of being overwhelmed. With fewer choices, less to clean, and less to organize, you are giving yourself a gift of freedom with more opportunities to connect with others, nature, and yourself.

Do the Maintenance

Inspect and clean your home regularly. Take care of minor repairs and problems before they snowball. A leaky faucet wastes ten thousand gallons of water a year! Get into the habit of tending to your home's needs as soon as they arise. An unchanging, ongoing to-do list drains your psyche, and a shabby, unclean home magnetizes lethargy.

Need some motivation? Start with clearing off a few surfaces and do a quick collection and return of misplaced items. Completing these easy, yet high-impact tasks can spur on tackling more industrious accomplishments.

Balanced Decorating

A balance in eco-friendly decorating—just as in life—is essential, as we learned in the previous chapter. If you are already acquiring your sustainable décor from under a hundred-mile radius of your home, look into some accent pieces from fair trade cooperatives. If your furniture is mostly recycled, repurposed, and reused, indulge in fresh bed linens and towels that are made from bamboo or organic cotton. Under the wide range of eco-friendly home goods, there are many possibilities that offer you a variety of choices to create a dynamic and balanced home.

SPIRITUAL SUSTAINABILITY

Your chosen home and the karmic lessons encased within those walls along the way are all a part of your spiritual journey. A spiritually supportive home feeds your soul, enhances personal growth, and inexplicably feels "right" to all who visit and live there.

"Goodwill" Decorating

When you choose paint made from organic flaxseed or linseed oil that is solvent free, you are making deliberate choices for greater wellness. When you choose pure fabrics such as silk, linen, jute, or hemp over synthetics, your home feels breathable and natural. When you buy furniture that has been gently used, you are giving it a second life and not being another cog in the consumer wheel that burdens the planet. Each one of these healthier, mindful choices generates a thriving, vibrant atmosphere in your home.

Minimize Electronics

You learned about the harmful effects of electronic pollution on your body in chapter 7. Here is how it can cause havoc on your psyche: too many televisions in a home diminish opportunities for spiritual connectivity. To start with, avoid televisions in all bedrooms. Electronic activity before bed reduces your ability to get a peaceful night's sleep, so get into new habits of reading a real page-turner rather than a tablet and avoid charging your phone and laptop near the bed. By lightening your electronic load, you are decreasing energy use and increasing conscious living.

Home Axis

For many, the epicenter of their home is the kitchen. For others, it's their garden. For some, it's the dining table where loved ones gather. Wherever the heart of your home may be, it is the foundation for what matters most to you. This sacred hub is the best place to introduce sustainability in new and creative ways. For example, if the kitchen is your focus, brainstorm how to make the most of composting with your family (no composter? Freeze scraps and when convenient, deliver to a community garden or farmers' market) or formulating inventive recipes from leftovers. If your garden is your glory, think of what part of your bounty can be donated to a soup kitchen or family in need. Intimate, environmental acts formed in your comfort zone will be the most genuine and effective on a global scale.

Reflect on House Karma

Have you ever thought about what brought you to your current home and the events that led up to you ending up in this space? Being that your home can be your teacher, what has your journey taught you? Has it been a rough road of renovations that reminded you to expect the unexpected and that patience is key? Did you trade in an urban life for a country setting because you realized you wanted a quieter, greener quality of life? Whether it's work relocation, a better school system, economics, downsizing, or weather preferences, the possibilities are endless, yet the lessons are all encoded. You are in your home, your community, your city, your state for a reason, and it doesn't matter if it's been three years or thirty, your space and the journey that led you to it right now has affected who you are. Think about the circumstances that led you to your current home. If you had to sum it up in one word, would it be luck? Intuition? Desperation? Then, try to connect how that theme carries over to other areas of your life.

If it's a negative situation—for example, bankruptcy forced you to find another place to live—reflect on what that has taught you. Then, intentionally bring in a new counterbalance by simplifying your belongings and focusing on cultivating the energy of abundance into your space.

CASE STUDY: BEA JOHNSON, AUTHOR OF *ZERO WASTE HOME*

Bea Johnson likes to reflect on a quote from Gandhi regarding her sustainable living. "Gandhi once said: 'Happiness is when what you think, what you say, and what you do are in harmony.' The Zero Waste lifestyle has done exactly that for us. Our home testifies that our lives are based on experiences instead of things, that our time is focused on relationships versus home maintenance. Voluntary simplicity has improved our lives so much, brought us closer as a family, and made us so much happier that we could not envision going back to the way we used to live!"

Voluntary simplicity is for me the most rewarding and enriching aspect of the zero waste lifestyle. Letting go was so easy that the challenge became knowing where to stop!

The dining room (on the next page) is Johnson's favorite part of the home. "It's open to the kitchen, it's the liveliest part of our home. In the evening, this is where we do homework, collaborate on projects, discuss the kids' grades, eat, drink, converse, laugh, cry, and sometimes yell—I have two teenage boys.

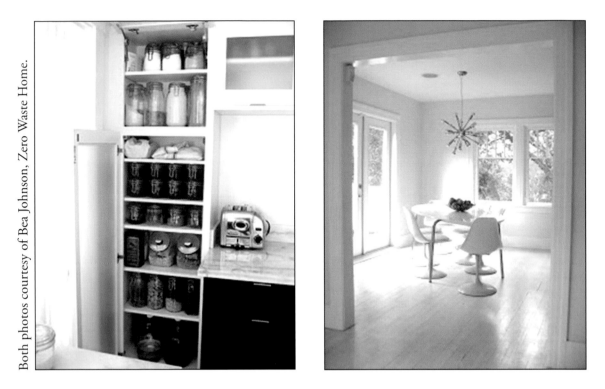

Both photos courtesy of Bea Johnson, Zero Waste Home.

"Each night, we each share what we're grateful for. This is also where I am most comfortable working during the day. It is surrounded by windows, which we keep uncovered to let the outdoors in. On summer days, I open the adjacent French doors, and it instantly becomes part of the outdoors. Squirrels and all kinds of birds, such as hummingbirds and blue jays, come by to say hello: They give me the strength to keep fighting for natural conservation and spread the zero waste lifestyle."

HOLISTIC SUSTAINABILITY IN YOUR BACKYARD

Creating a Garden of Intention

Step out your back door and a whole new world of possibilities and opportunities to enhance your garden *and your life* await you. In addition to the sustainable aspects of composting, rainwater collection, and growing your own food, holistic sustainability draws upon ancient connections between nature and yourself from a physical, emotional, and spiritual perspective. By applying these principles to your own life, your backyard is no longer just a separate outdoor area behind the house. It becomes a dedicated ground for consecrating goals—both in landscape and in life—while acknowledging nature and allowing the best to unfold.

Begin by shifting your perspective. In your mind's eye, see your garden as a fertile plot that allows you to manifest your desires in symbolic representations. Want more prosperity in your life? Imagine the bountiful energy that is cultivated from a yard full of growing, vibrant life forces that are alive with chi. That abundant energy force, especially if it has been conceived and cultivated by your own head, heart, and hands, creates a supportive foundation for a continuous flow of prosperity and opportunity. By your purposely planting and nourishing plant life while making connections to whatever your goals may be, your garden takes on new intention and a deeper meaning.

Mind

Ask Yourself, What Are My Garden Goals?

Be clear with your vision and know your needs. Do you want a quaint nook where you can relax with a cup of tea? Do you need a dynamic and lively space to entertain? Would you love to have a spot to cultivate your own food? Do you envision a maintenance-free garden? Do you dream about having a horticulture showplace? A killer composting system? Imagine your ideal backyard in specific detail.

Plan Ahead

Create a visual board with pictures clipped from magazines and catalogs. Look for images you would want in your ideal backyard. Include key words that exemplify your desires. As you do this process, visualize that you are also "sowing the seeds" of your related goals (i.e., relaxation, recognition, sustenance).

Body

Conduct an Exploration

Make a clean sweep through your garden in its current state. Remove dead foliage, weeds, and debris while visualizing the removal of negative energy in your life that no longer serves you. Let that bag of dead weeds represent something specific—like negative relationships, excessive worry, or self-doubt—as you remove it from your space.

Be Present in the Moment

As your backyard takes shape, document the changes with photos, a video, or in a journal. Take pride in your accomplishments and the transformations that have occurred, however big or small they might be.

A projector makes outlining a lotus image in chalk very easy. Afterward a tube of pink acrylic paint fills it in, and less than an hour later, the backyard is transformed.

Spirit

Become a Visionary

When you fertilize the soil, envision that you are adding a catalyst of support to your visual goal board. As you water and nourish your garden, you are also cultivating your life goals. As you add symbols that you resonate with, like the lotus above, you are creating a visual inspiration for your goals.

Reap What You Sow

Since energy goes where attention flows, your rewards will become tantamount to your efforts. Where roots take hold, flowers and plants abound. Parlay that energy of accomplishment to your life goals. Sometimes growth won't occur, but where it does,

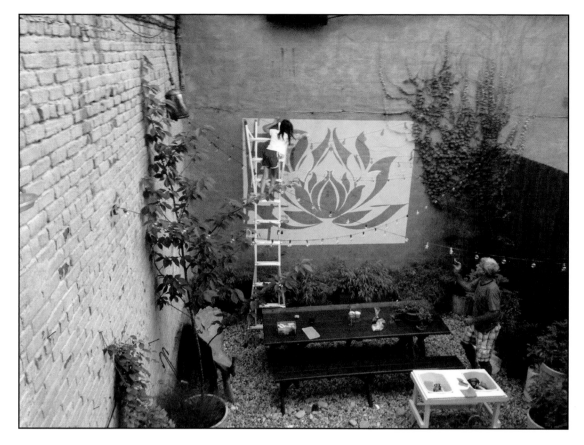

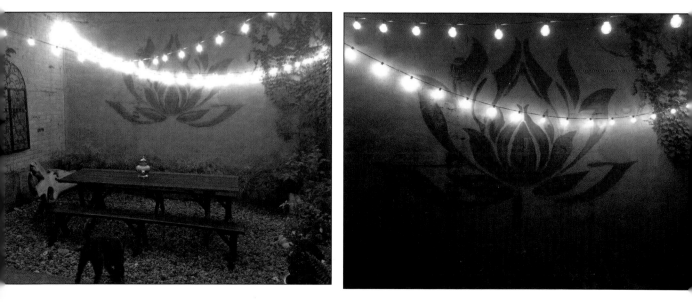

focus on the life force of success visually taking hold in front of you. By doing so, you reinforce the same powerful message in your daily life.

Using the Elements in Your Garden

Wood, Fire, Earth, Metal, and Water are essential energies in our garden that can initiate profound change in and around us. Intentionally tapping into these energies can transform your yard and improve your personal goals in numerous ways.

Recognition with the Fire Element

Use the element Fire with actual fire; such as a chiminea, candles, torches, a barbecue grill, a fire pit, or with lighting. Another option is using the color red in your plantings.

By adding red flowers to your garden you can tap into the fire energy, which in turn enhances your fame and recognition. Whether you are focusing on perfecting a batch of tomatoes or cultivating a prize rose garden, use this color in your yard while visualizing your fame, reputation, and integrity flourishing too.

Relaxation with the Water Element

Water features can be a very effective addition in providing a sense of balance and well-being to your yard. The water element enhances wealth, spirituality, and inspiration. It can

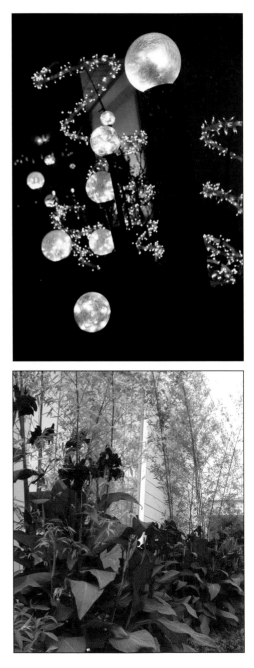

also help clarify your thinking. Make sure the water is clean and flowing gracefully. Stagnant or murky water is similar to stuck energy and will impede the flow in your life. If you have ponds, bays, or streams in your backyard, try to make the most of them by situating seating and visual interest toward the water element.

Communication with the Metal Element

Metal assists in opening up the lines of communication. Wrought-iron patio furniture, fencing, or metal sculptures are ways to bring in this element. When purchasing and placing these outdoor metal items, focus your intention on enhancing relationships of all kinds—friendships, community, work, love, and family.

Stability with Earth Element

Terra-cotta planters, pottery, brick, and ceramics are all ways you can bring solidity to a chaotic environment. If your backyard is in the midst of a busy city, near a fast-moving highway, or swift-moving water, bring in the Earth element for its stabilizing effect. The same is true if your lifestyle is chaotic or you are going through times of uncertainty. Rock gardens, stone borders, and brick pathways bring in a deep sense of stability and foundation. A boulder-size rock can also have the same effect by adding a symbolic point of strength and solidness to your land.

Growth with the Wood Element

Energetically, this element fosters intuition, creativity, expansion, and growth. It is found in plants, flowers, and wooden outdoor furniture. Wooden window boxes, decks, and railroad ties are also useful options for this element. Since most outdoor spaces are filled with the wood element already, try to focus your intention on specific areas of interest that you desire growth in. For example, when planting a tree, there are many benefits to acknowledge (beautifying the landscape, adding oxygen to the environment, creating a sound barrier), but also focus on a personal goal such as "this tree represents our first home purchase and new beginnings filled with hope and gratitude." Imparting a silent blessing while you are cultivating your wish dovetails the intention and the corporeal energy together.

We know that humankind energetically syncopates in conjunction with nature. In chapter 3, we discussed the cyclical examples nature and Man share. A garden is a perfect microcosm of the Earth's continuous cycles. There are countless ways a growing garden can at times symbolize events, issues, or challenges in our life and become our fertile teacher. Growth and abundance is the Yang cousin to the essential Yin force of restraint and patience. When communities or businesses become rapidly overdeveloped without a system of checks and balances, energies can get out of control, identity can get lost, focus or disruptions can occur. With gardening, a balance comes in the form of pruning, weeding, clearing out debris, and clipping. By way of pruning, each cut has the potential to change the growth of the tree. Focus is required before mindfully making a cut. A client told me a story about how she was dreading having to fire an employee at her job. Days leading up to it, she would sit in her garden and contemplate the how and when of the much-needed task. "It was my apple tree that gave me insight. There was crowding at the crown and some branches were starting to look diseased. The tree's growth was dependent on necessary cutting. I didn't realize at first that this was the one spot that I would come to contemplate the firing decision. Then one day, it came to me how, like the pruning of the tree, the decision to cut the employee would ultimately end up helping not only my company but change her trajectory for the better in the long run."

Choosing Moving or Still Water

Water can be added in two energy states: moving or still. Flowing, active, and circulating water can be found in outdoor fountains or landscaped waterfalls. Dynamic and flowing water helps you have a strong circulating cash flow. Still water can be found in a tabletop bowl of water, a birdbath, ponds, lakes, or pools. Still water represents accumulated wealth. When your water feature is clean and clear, it symbolizes a calm state of mind and financial clarity. When it is dirty and murky, it represents stagnant finances and a lack of opportunities.

By tuning into nature and the elements that surround you, you can transform your backyard into a visually rewarding and sacred place that will help create the life you desire. Know that your participation from conception to fruition has allowed it to happen.

HOLISTIC SUSTAINABILITY IN YOUR COMMUNITY

Now that you've stepped outside of your home to the backyard, keep it going and look around at your community. Are there areas that could be improved? Could you use a community watch, slower speed limits, "No Littering" signs, a farmers' market, bike lanes, or more trees planted? There are always ways that neighborhoods can be improved. Here are ten basic steps that can help speed the process along and make a difference.

1. ***Start a Listserv.*** Once you have a means for communication in place, connecting about everything from break-ins to block parties is easy. One email to the list alerts everyone on it.
2. ***Form a moniker.*** If you don't already have one, create a name for your neighborhood group. A name could be a fusion of the streets that form it, the official block association name, or a play on words of the larger neighborhood it is from. A name creates your identity and helps get plans of action under way.
3. ***Have meetings.*** Neighborhood meetings ignite conversations and can get the ball rolling for area challenges.
4. ***Go with the flow.*** Park in the right direction. Nothing diminishes the energy and feel of a neighborhood quicker than parking against the flow of traffic. In suburban towns (this wouldn't happen in major cities) when residents choose to park in front of their home in this manner, it greatly lowers the vibration of the area. Against-the-flow parking creates a subconscious feeling of chaos, neglect, confusion, and laziness.

5. ***Seek sponsorship.*** You might be surprised how many big-box home improvement stores are amenable to sponsoring a Clean Up and Planting Day for your organization. Some retailers may offer a one-time-only deep discount in their garden center. It's a great opportunity to get what's needed for clearing out an abandoned lot and making it into a community garden or for transforming neighborhood tree pits.

6. ***Create continuity.*** If you have an issue with getting people to clean up after their dogs or to stop littering, consider creating waterproof signs you hang around the trees that ask people to curb their dogs and not litter. Make it personal ("We are working hard trying to keep our neighborhood clean"), and be sure to include a thank-you for doing so by your neighborhood group name.

7. ***Get connected.*** Get to know your community affairs officer, local precinct, and politicians so that when you need action, you are familiar with each other and have a larger network in seeking resolutions.

8. ***Plant.*** A tree-lined block has a higher property value than a barren one. Besides the majestic beauty and shade offerings, trees help clean pollutants from the air.

9. ***Get to know your neighbors.*** Make an effort to do more than an obligatory "Hi, how are you?" If you are even somewhat close with your neighbor, they can look out for your property, take your deliveries when you're not there, or lend you a tool when you need it. It's worth it.

10. ***Be kind and be aware.*** When you are sharing walls (brownstones, apartments, condominiums, etc.), dwell with consideration, give a heads-up if you are having a party, and don't let your dog bark excessively.

MY STORY: HOME IS WHERE THE . . . EMOTIONAL SUSTAINABILITY IS

When guests come in and ask if they should take off their shoes, I say, "However you are comfortable." And I mean it. (Unless they had severely dirty boots, dripping with mud, then I'd say "Sure, let's get 'em off. Here's some slippers!") Like many other people, I want my home to be a relaxed and comfortable gathering place for good times with friends and loved ones, yet I also prefer it to be clean and somewhat orderly.

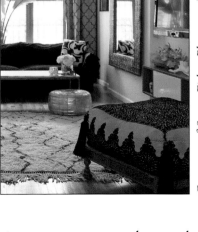

My white Beni Ourain Moroccan rug in a high-traffic spot exemplifies that concept. It's thick and fluffy, made by hand with meaning in the Atlas mountains, and serves as a cushy hub for all kinds of family activities. The best part is, I can just take it to the self-serve laundry and stuff it into the giant triple loader. Maybe that's not the proper way to clean a fine rug, but it comes out super clean and afterward I feel nice and fluffy too! I am one of those people who, when I have a clean home, it makes me feel good.

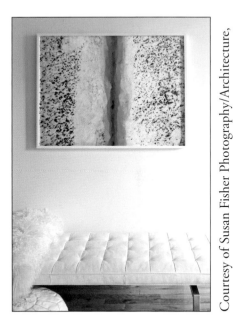

I strive for the "in between" spot throughout my home—treasured items that hold meaning but are not so precious that we are living precariously and treading lightly. I aim for comfortable furnishings and rugs, but not so sloppy and beat-up that the energy of the house feels neglected and dirty. Stains, smudged walls, torn furnishings, and piles of papers all exude a lower energy and bring you down. On the other end of the spectrum are overly curated spaces that look like an excessively staged photo shoot where every angle has been analyzed and labored over. (How many interior design photo shoots will continue to place the ubiquitous designer high heels artfully tossed on the floor of the closet or next to the bed? It's so contrived.)

Besides the fluffy white wool rug that takes a beating, I have a white leather modern bench that I clean with a dry-erase sponge to remove marks. My black couch

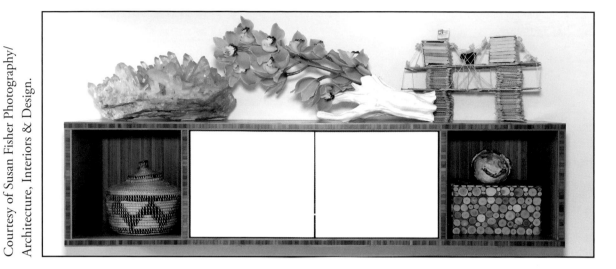

cushion covers easily zip off and can be thrown in my washing machine. It doesn't matter if wine, coffee, or throw up have landed here (all of which have occurred), cleanup is easy, and they are back to new quickly. My reclaimed teak Tuscan farm table takes the biggest hit of all with daily meals, writing, and art projects galore, yet the weathering adds to its lovely patina like a gracefully aging Italian actress who looks more beautiful with time. Because I know these heavily used items can be so forgiving, I am not anxious and freaked out when life happens in our active home. A low-maintenance, thoughtful home creates contentment and happiness in your space. Having highly used items that can clean well will give you peace of mind, which is priceless. Think of that when you make purchases for items like these.

Creating rituals or meaningful habits inside your home is a great way to honor and care for your space and self, while also increasing emotional sustainability. These rituals don't have to be drenched in religious dogma or new age fodder; just make it a regular routine that feels special and positive. Before we eat, we gather hands and say what we are thankful for. This action is simple and easy to do and will always increase moods and the energy of the space rather quickly. Almost daily I light incense. To me, it always makes the home feel grounded and the energy in the home clean.

I also tap into the emotional and spiritual properties of essential oils and use them daily in a diffuser. I love changing up the blends according to our needs. When we need to wind down, it's lavender, chamomile, and sandalwood. Need to focus and enhance memory? I choose grapefruit, rosemary, and frankincense. I love using the top citrus notes for an energy boost and the deeper base notes for grounding and contemplation. Each family member enjoys picking scents according to their needs. Whether it's habits to generate gratitude or ones that stimulate and guide the senses, rituals can be balm to your psyche and help create a home that deeply supports you.

An emotionally sustainable home isn't compared to other spaces for what it does or does not have. If you come from that mind-set, your home will never be enough, and flaws, lack of space, bad layout, and so forth will feed into a growing discontent that fills up *you and your home.* If you can't renovate or make changes, it is important to accept your space with its shortcomings and focus on the positive features. When a home has served its purpose, but over time needs have changed, there comes a time to move on. Read Sue's story below for more.

CASE STUDY: SUE INGEBRETSON'S ANAHEIM HILLS, CALIFORNIA, HOME

Sue Ingebretson is one of the top experts in fibromyalgia, and she is aware of how sensitive a body can be to its environment. Her husband built their home with Sue's holistic

health care practice, RebuildingWellness. com, in mind. The gardens are organic, the water system uses potassium instead of chemical-based salts, and a courtyard fountain taps into the soothing sounds of gurgling water that you can enjoy from every room in the house. She hosts weekly tai chi classes in her home as well

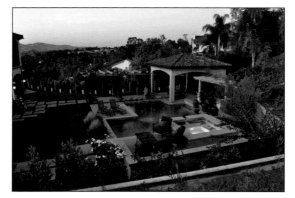

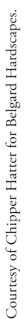

Courtesy of Chipper Hatter for Belgard Hardscapes.

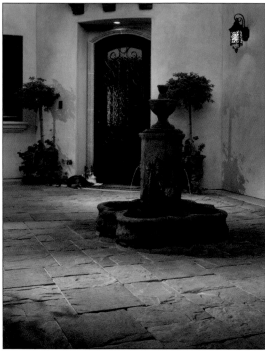

as healthy cooking classes that infuse her home with beneficial and healing chi. Her dog, Pup, seen in this photo at the front door, "sets the energy" of the house by tuning in to what is needed in the moment by those inside. She calls her kitchen the heart of the home and her courtyard, the soul. "I feel supported. My clients enjoy this respite from their busy lives when they come to see me. I've heard them say that my home is an oasis, or a little slice of paradise. I couldn't agree more." She moved into this home when she began a new cycle of her life as author of *FibroWHYalgia* and has been grateful for every day that she has spent here. The home has supported her journey with physical, emotional, and spiritual sustainability while her book became a best seller and she became a leading expert in this field. However, now she and her husband have outgrown the large space and are ready to find another "project" home they can make their own. I found Sue's progressive-minded rumination about the house to be both profound and admirable: "We've loved this house for a season and now it's time to begin another."

WHEN IT'S TIME TO MOVE

There is a reason why moving is considered one of the biggest stressors in a person's life, right up there with illness, divorce, and death. It is so much more than the physical drain of packing up your life in boxes or the mental strain of the logistics of it all. It's the emotional facets that can have the biggest impact on you. Whether you are thrilled to move on or filled with sadness that you are leaving, there is one very specific thing that will enable you to make the transition more effortless. It's saying a proper farewell to your home. (I never did this to my beloved childhood home in Milltown, New Jersey, and to this day, nearly two decades later, I still dream about it regularly, and every once in a while I nostalgically drive by it. I think the rest of my family feel I'm wistfully obsessive about it.)

When the time is close for leaving the home for good and you have a quiet moment by yourself, walk through each room. Recall the most prominent memories that occurred there, good or bad. Walk the perimeter of the property too. Spend as much time as you need. Thank the home for being the carousel to your memories and the protecting shelter for your loved ones. Send the home golden light that connects to you. As you turn and walk away, let the light remain with the house and slowly disconnect from you. Surround yourself with a new, brighter light. Say good-bye. Look forward.

If throughout this book you have been able to make the connections to yourself and your space and have begun setting up your home with mind, body, and spirit awareness, you might be asking yourself, *Now what? I'm feeling good, I'm reaching goals, I'm organized.* You may have even begun to notice how other people's spaces are mirroring their issues. Now it's time to take what you've learned and examine how other environments can affect you and discover what you can learn from them.

CHAPTER NINE

Holistic Excellence: When It All Comes Together (or Not) in People, Places, and Things

"If you look for perfection, you'll never be content."

—Leo Tolstoy

Whether it's the products we use or the places we go, when all factors of mind, body, and spirit thoughtfully unite, you may feel an extraordinary difference. Healing can occur more rapidly, goals can be realized more effusively, and relaxation can be achieved more wholly. Products that are consciously made may feel meaningful and more effective. By now, your awareness is most likely heightened in your own home, so let's take those principles further. When you venture outside your home to appointments, shopping, vacations, how are you affected by these spaces? Could the waiting room atmosphere at your doctor's office be enhancing your anxiety? What makes one luxury Caribbean resort feel so much better than a similar one elsewhere? Would your shopping experience feel different if it was done in an environment that considered nearly every holistic detail? Here are some examples of spaces that fall short and need some tweaking, as well as examples of when it all comes together in a thoroughly comprehensive way. Grasp these details and you'll discover how you can better handle your own mistakes more effectively in order to achieve your personal best in all areas of your life.

A NEW YORK CITY HOSPITAL: WAITING FOR IMPROVEMENT

This book began with my diagnosis and has spanned fourteen years. During that time, I've logged quite a few hours in the waiting room of a New York City hospital's cancer treatment center that will have to remain unnamed. Through the years, the cancer center has been moved around throughout the hospital, growing to an entire wing and eventually into its own brand-new building. On one particular visit when a nurse asked me what my occupation was and then how I felt about the energy of this hospital's new center, I immediately rattled off a few points that I felt could be improved. I was then given the contact information of the patient care coordinator, who was hired to work on and improve these exact aspects of a patient's experience. Below are just a few of my points in my assessment that I sent to her.

When patients arrive for appointments, they are most likely already anxious, stressed, and ill at ease. Patient waiting areas need to be particularly tended to for their cleanliness, efficiency, warmth, and comfort levels. This can be most effectively addressed by looking at subconscious influences in design and symbolic elements in both the bigger picture and the details of the environment. Most notable challenges in the new center are that it feels cold and impersonal with all the sleek surfaces and vast stonework.

- Currently, the entrance and waiting areas feel lifeless and austere. A symbolic design element that offers vibrancy and a vital sense of flourishing life would be the use of live foliage. Due to the contamination concerns for the patients who have immune compromised issues, there are options that can be looked into that do not need dirt, pesticides, or fertilizer. Bamboo is naturally antibacterial and antifungal as well as being naturally resistant to mildew. Bamboo is also low-maintenance. Placed in a bed of smooth river rocks with up lighting, it can be a stunning design element in the waiting room on either side of the main signage. The current sunlight at that location is sufficient for the bamboo.

- Televisions in the waiting area should play either a loop of the hospital's messages, functions, and reminders, or pleasing nature-related material on a continuous loop, not daytime talk shows or twenty-four-hour news channels. The latter two are not conducive to relaxation and serenity, and mostly promote negativity and subconsciously heighten anxiety.

- A water element would significantly help alter the austerity of the environment. Upon entering the building, a water wall in the waiting area would help. A saltwater aquarium would also be an option. Studies have shown that watching an underwater scene significantly reduces blood pressure. Listening to waterfall sounds are soothing and relaxing.

- Artwork is needed to warm up the space. To bring in community, consider a rotating "gallery" of artwork from local artists. This could be a mutually beneficial agreement of no or minimal cost. Rotation every eight to ten weeks promotes a sense of freshness. Consider artwork such as tabletop sculptures for the coffee tables in the waiting room. Make sure that the subconscious symbolism in the artwork is uplifting, inspiring, and beautiful. Any artwork that is shocking and provocative is not ideal here.

- Consider bringing in decorative items for the coffee tables that provide interest and a sense of "home" and "comfort." While this emotion is subjective, there are items that can universally warm up the space and provide a point of interest for conversation or reflection. Replace the tattered and dated magazines with beautiful coffee table books. Also, fun objects of distraction could be considered, such as mechanical and logic puzzles.

- Offer aromatherapy packets on some tables in the waiting area for patients who are interested. These individual wipes of various natural scents can aid in the frustrations and anxiety levels for the patients; for example, lemon uplifts, lavender relaxes, and tea tree oil purifies.

- Care-related factors such as Patient Services are crucial in the overall hospital experience (according to *U.S. News & World Report* criteria in ranking the best hospitals). Favorable patient experiences cannot be underestimated. When a patient arrives in the waiting area, there needs to be more hands-on care and attention to detail during the check-in process.

- All litter should be removed from the check-in desks. While patients are going through the check-in process, they are staring at both the back of two mounted computer screens and whatever garbage—crumpled papers, drink cups, and so forth—is left out on the desktop. Diligence is needed here to promote a sense of order and cleanliness.

- More care should be taken to pronounce patient names correctly. Also, when hospital employees come out to call a patient in to their appointment, consider developing a system of identification beforehand. It is distracting when a name is called loudly over and over and a search ensues around the waiting area for this person.

- Water for patients should be provided. A stand or table with water coolers that have lemon or cucumber available is a small investment with a big value. It creates a wellness-like atmosphere and underscores the importance of health and hydration.

I never received feedback from my assessment (just confirmation that they received it) and a few months later found out the patient care coordinator was no longer there. Nearly one year later, none of my suggestions was implemented. At my most recent appointment, I had to wait for two hours before my blood was even tested, standing the whole time because there was not enough seating. This was followed by an additional hour in a treatment room waiting for the doctor. I'm certain the hospital is thriving, but I also know that the overall patient experience could be improved.

Motivated by a similar need for holistic improvements in hospitals, fashion designer and philanthropist Donna Karan founded Urban Zen, a charitable organization that aims to change the present healthcare paradigm by addressing wellness issues with their integrative therapy program. Their program is now implemented in the Ronald

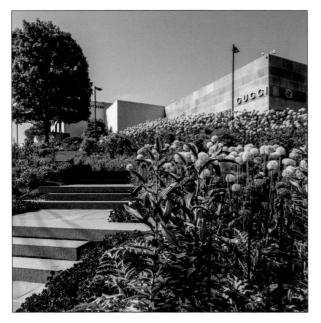

Reagan UCLA Medical Center where Eastern healing techniques are offered with yoga, breath awareness, Reiki, essential oil therapy, and nutrition. Karan's pioneering approach of acknowledging the importance of Western medicine yet also seeing the necessity of healing that "can only be accessed from the heart and through the spirit" is creating a new model of holistic wellness and patient care in hospitals that is greatly needed.

AMERICANA MANHASSET: A HOLISTIC RETAIL WONDERLAND

Americana Manhasset, in Long Island, New York, is a premier shopping location where high-end retailers such as Gucci, Bottega Veneta, Cartier, Chanel, Hermès, Fendi, Prada, and many others reside. But it is not just the impressive collection of stores, which feature an elevated level of excellence in goods and customer service, that makes this shopping destination so spectacular. It is also not just that Oehme van Sweden syncopates the landscape designs with seasonal palettes that reflect the liveliness of the cyclical fashions, or even that renowned architect Peter Marino oversees every square foot of development to ensure continuity. What makes this location so spectacular is the meticulous attention to every detail of the shopper's experience. And your experience starts even before you arrive. The Americana Manhasset has sponsored roadway beautification for some of the surrounding roads leading up to the entrance, which gradually builds an imperceptible feel of community stewardship and goodwill that continues as you get closer with each step.

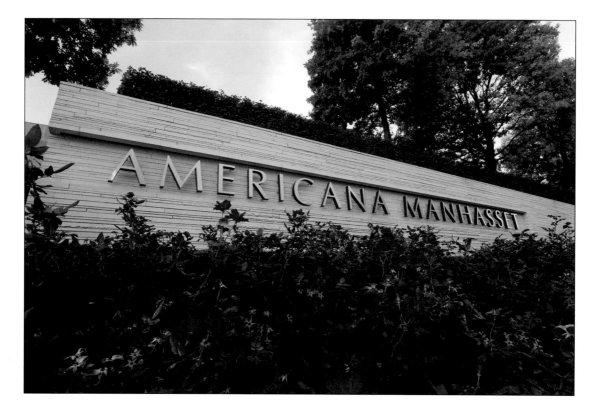

The entrance organically welcomes you with wispy, native Long Island sea grasses and thriving foliage, while dynamic water features are found at the ends of two landscaped walkways. Even the garbage cans are beautiful. These sleek, metal splendors were found in Europe by hands-on owner Frank Castagna himself. You might think that with such luxurious brands and a meticulously considered environment there would be a supercilious air permeating the premises, but the opposite is true, and that is what it is so special. For example, Americana Personal Shopper Danielle Merollo's genuine down-to-earth helpfulness and ability to read people is refreshing. ("You already have two similar ones in your closet," she once said to an undecided regular customer.) Like Frank Castagna on the corporate level, Danielle helps set the tone at the store level, which is one of inclusiveness, comfort, and warmth.

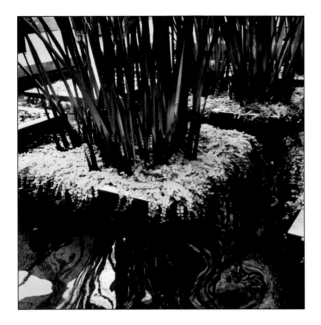

Diversity is on the forefront with interpreters on hand at the concierge to assist foreign shoppers and directories nearby to guide them. I asked Senior Vice President and Creative Director Andrea Sanders, "What is the one thing that people would be most surprised to learn about the Americana?" She replied, "How much we really listen and respond to the needs of the community," and added that their various initiatives have organically grown by doing so. Champions for Charity, Americana's

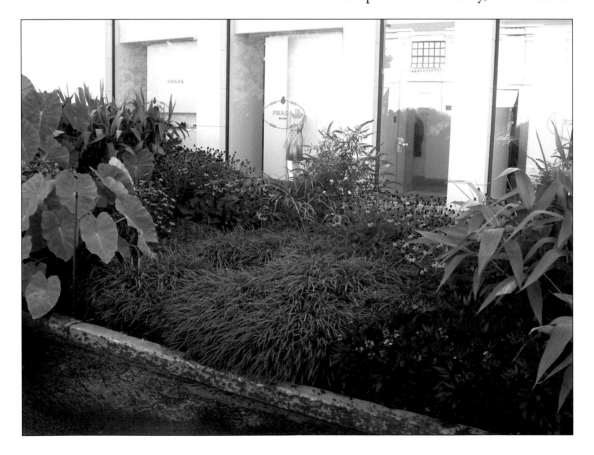

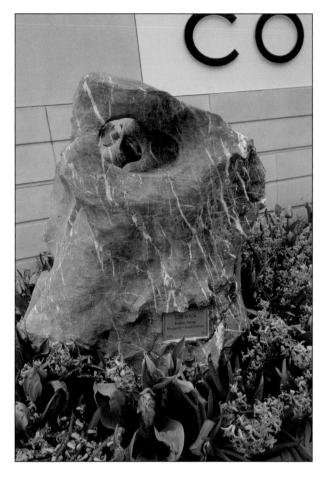

annual holiday shopping benefit, is a great example of that responsiveness to the community, as shoppers can make purchases knowing the nonprofit of their choice (from over one hundred charities) will greatly benefit with each purchase. There is also Americana's ongoing support of Northwell Health, which includes many hospitals and wellness programs in the area. A major fall fashion show raises significant funds for women's health initiatives in particular.

Holistic excellence happens here because from the moment you enter, you are greatly welcomed and enveloped in a higher vibrational atmosphere of understated yet highly considered precision. Americana does not broadcast its levels of altruism and the magnitude of their attention to detail. You get to discover that on your own as you stroll around and find such blithe surprises as the Life Rock, also known as the Prosperity Good Luck Rock. The customer service is sincere because there is no annoying pressure. Each boutique-like structure is physically masterful and reflects the exceptional goods inside them. All aspects of this thriving, thoughtful atmosphere come together in an experiential expression that, simply put, leaves you feeling good. If you get a chance, go rub the lucky prosperity rock on the property. As this place is filled with so much good juju, hopefully you can take a little bit of it home with you.

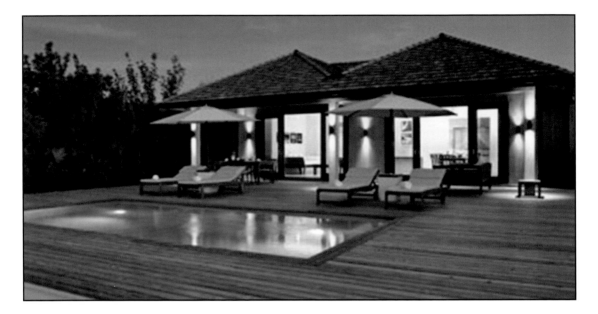

HOLISTIC EXCELLENCE: COMO PARROT CAY TURKS AND CAICOS

When I went to Parrot Cay in Turks and Caicos, I was blown away. I was enveloped in the understated superfluity of the COMO Hotels and Resorts experience. You can find glowing reviews online that go into every outstanding detail and easily understand why it was voted the #1 Hotel in the Caribbean by *Condé Nast Traveler*, *Elite Traveler*, and also *Travel + Leisure*, and I agree with every single accolade it has been given, but I am going to share with you a specific characteristic that takes Parrot Cay above and beyond the many other resorts that herald themselves with the overused "luxury" label and the ways Parrot Cay deeply connects all the right dots.

The nature of what I do leads me to notice elements in my surroundings, from grand to subtle. Sometimes on vacation this is a curse, as instead of fully relaxing, I might be mentally making a list of ways things can be improved. And other rare times, like at Parrot Cay, I am awed by the attention to detail, outstanding professionalism,

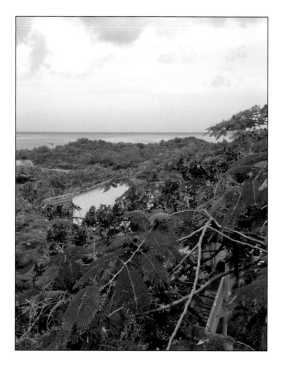

and—here's the reason I am writing about them—their humbleness. It shows up in ways that are simultaneously over the top and under the radar.

Signs and loud consumer packaging are subliminal visual clutter. There is a lack of unnecessary signage that pervades the resort experience, which allows the pure beauty of the environment and the journey of discovery to take center stage. This enables the resort to present like a humble friend with quiet confidence whose beautiful attributes you discover as they unfold over time.

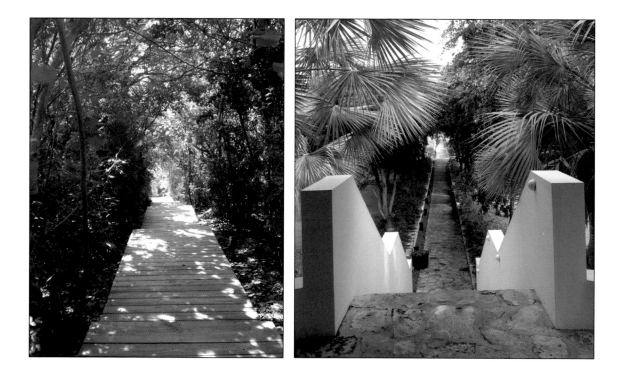

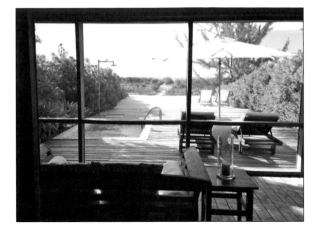

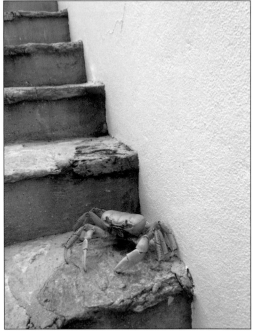

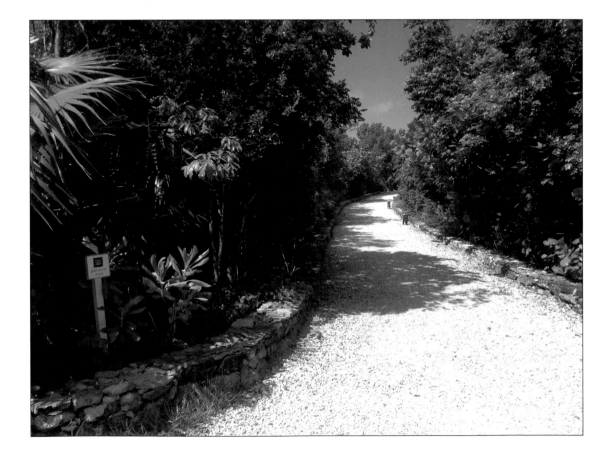

From the unmarked front entrance of the resort to the screened-in hut (below) overlooking the marsh that my husband and I found just by chance during a long walk—there is such joy in unanticipated discovery.

One morning, my husband took a jog back to that isolated, unmarked hut and was surprised to see that an employee was there tidying up and uncovering the daybed that had been covered up the night before. Who knows if any other guests even found that hut while I stayed there—but there it was, just waiting to be found and ready to accommodate whoever might encounter it. Walkways throughout the resort have no signage either, but when it's absolutely necessary, like the beach houses, villas, or the spa, you'll find it, tastefully and discreetly showing you the way.

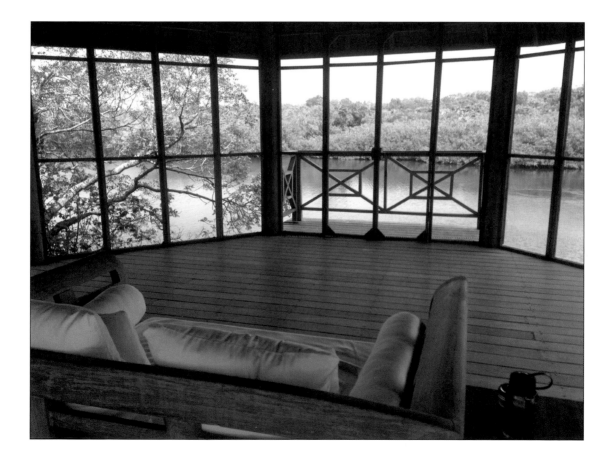

The physical attributes come in the form of inconspicuous design details and services that are simultaneously extravagant and inconspicuous. Whenever I noticed a clever design detail—whether it was a folded reading light on the nightstand or a conveniently placed shelf next to the claw-foot tub to hold shampoo or a wine glass, I was told it was the design detail brilliance of Don Diaz. When I first met the dapper fellow who manages the beach houses and villas, he was checking the perimeter of one of the absolutely incredible two-bedroom beach villas in anticipation of the new arrivals. Just making sure that everything looked up to par, I suppose. He modestly smiled as I gushed about his thoughtful insights and told me he "watches a lot of HGTV."

The spiritual aspects occur with how the land is honored and the resort is laid out. The land and the guests are greatly respected in Parrot Cay. General Manager Grant Noble's admirable dedication to honoring the land (according to an employee, he won't allow any of the indigenous trees to be cut down—even if it were to open up a coveted ocean view) is as powerful as his dedication to every guest, for whom he leaves a handwritten personal greeting upon room arrival. Recyclable water bottles are left on each nightstand, nature walks are available, and a palm tree planting and naming project from last Christmas ensures a lower carbon footprint with a personalized twist.

The layout of the resort is in alignment with the energetic flow of the surrounding land, which further enhances an inexplicable feeling that everything "just feels right." Candles are strategically placed throughout rooms and even at the front desk, which greatly adds to a glowing, inviting atmosphere of warmth.

Your subconscious picks up on subtle cues—whether it is an imbalanced waiting room or a well-thought-out shopping or vacation destination. Granted, a cancer treatment waiting room in the hospital is not a fun excursion like shopping or an island vacation, where people are in completely different states of mind and conditions. But that is precisely why it's all the more reason for places where stress or tension naturally reside (like the workplace, airports, and hospitals) to take their prompts from the places that get it right. When you are in a vulnerable state, you need your environment to step it up even more. When specific details of mind, body, spirit, and space all connect together to provide a holistic encounter, you will be in a more open and aware state to fulfill your aims of that location.

MY STORY: CREATING THE HOLISTIC HOME COMPANY— PERFECTION IN IMPERFECTION

At Christmas 2013, my eight-year-old daughter, Luchia, and I wanted to make all of our gifts for friends and family. We started with what we knew well and use often: candles and body scrubs. Besides perfecting the product with many test runs, we really got into the presentation, making labels and even brochures. We came up with a name—Brooklyn Apothecary—and locally sourced most of our ingredients, jars, and packaging materials. We researched the highest quality aromatherapy oils and customized each scrub or candle scent according to what we thought each person would need and enjoy. An aunt with hormone imbalances received geranium in her salt scrub; grapefruit helped another loved one feel rejuvenated; jasmine and lavender calmed another. Feedback was positive. When a friend said, "You know, you should really think about making these and selling them!" my reaction was to laugh. "I don't have time for that. I have a book to finish writing . . . classes to teach . . . clients to see and my family to enjoy." I didn't give it another thought. It seemed like an out of reach goal that I wasn't the least bit interested in.

A few months passed, and by chance, I was in a development deal for my own television show. I had hosted television segments before, but this was something potentially much bigger yet also something I could take or leave with equal measure. As it was getting shopped around to different networks, I was approached by some agents and management companies that were interested in representing me for talent and product branding. I went into one all-men-around-a-big-board-room-table meeting feeling awfully nervous, not knowing what to expect and not knowing exactly what I should say. But as the meeting went on, something happened I never even anticipated. I became unimpressed and disenchanted.

When I talked with the team about the growing trajectory of retail companies with a conscience that give back, like Warby Parker or Toms, they didn't grasp what I was referencing. When I asked questions about financial backing, retail industry connections, and distribution plans, there were no solid replies, only mumblings of one of their client's rock-star fame and signature hot sauce. I left feeling uninspired and never followed up. I am sure they felt the same way about me, because they never contacted me either.

The more I thought about that meeting afterward, the more I began to think, *Maybe I could try this on my own. I'll start small with a few items on a website.* I never would have considered this had it not been for that disappointing meeting. Whenever I contemplate taking a risk, my formula for action is simple. I always go through a worst-case scenario outcome. The worst I could come up with was that if this business failed, I would be out a nominal sum of money that would not break me, and then my friends and family would all receive some marvelous handmade gifts. The next two months were a whirlwind of coincidental events that propelled me to move forward in great leaps. As chapter 3 explains, when you *Get in Your Groove*, the Universe will help guide you along. That was what was occurring. Opportunities seemed to unfold effortlessly and with uncanny timing to push this new mission along. My online company of handmade luxury goods for the mind, body, spirit, and home was born. I named the business TheHolisticHomeCompany.com.

I live in Brooklyn, a fertile borough of creativity booming with innovative artisans and crafty makers at every corner. I began to collaborate with some, and we came up with beautiful, thoughtful, sustainable products to add to the collection. A talented sewer with a degree in textiles and I designed custom sheets. Small-business artisan, Stacy Hauger, who repurposes luxury fabrics, made the cosmetic and ditty bags. My custom aromatherapy goods offered customers the opportunity to pick their own top, middle, and base notes. This way, they could customize products based on their own scent preferences as well as their individual emotional and physical needs by tapping into what each different essential oil offered. Every product that The Holistic Home Company offers inspires your mind, revitalizes your body, stirs your soul, and enhances your home. Also, every single item is made while focusing on good thoughts so that customers can actually feel the goodness bursting from every product.

My right brain hated having to navigate my way through legal and financial necessities (who knew you had to announce your company in local newspapers for several weeks as one of the steps in forming an LLC, or the complexities of properly filing and categorizing your trademarks?), but somehow it all worked out. The aim of the company was that every product would be made with pure materials and be made while holding a positive intention

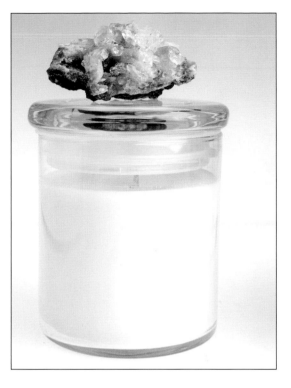

for the recipient. Like this book, every product would draw the associations to the importance of connecting mind, body, spirit, and space.

It's not just lighting a candle—it's taking a moment to pause, reflect, and gather an objective. For example, the candles are labeled like this:

Mind: Every time you light this candle, make a wish or hold a positive intention.

Body: All natural, pure soy wax with a cotton wick.

Spirit: In many cultures, a flame is symbolic of rituals, hope, reflection, and faith. Let this crystal candle symbolize your hopes and goals.

Space: Candles enhance the atmosphere with their golden illuminating glow. The attached crystal beautifies your surroundings.

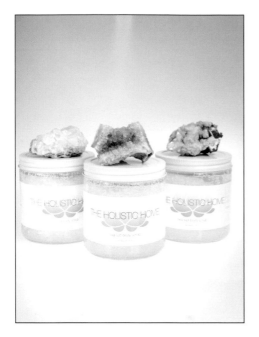

Visualizing getting rid of anything negative with each use of the sea salt body scrub was the "mind" tip. The all-natural, pure ingredients that leave your skin smooth and supple relate to the "body." The "spirit" portion is how you customize the top, middle, and base notes according to your own emotional needs by identifying the properties associated with each essential oil. Lastly, "space" relates to how every scrub comes with a one-of-a-kind crystal to enhance your surroundings.

Even the raw crystal napkin rings were encouraged to be used by "setting your positive intention as you set the table" as the mindful

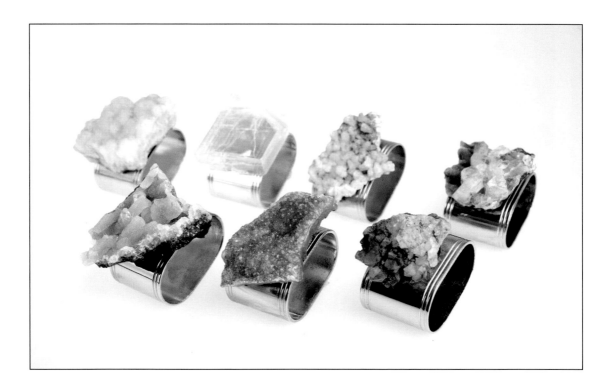

action tip. These crystal napkin rings were my pride and joy. I acquired the crystals from a sustainably mined family-run business in India and would often stare at them in wonderment at how nature had created these marvels. Every single one was different. As we turned them into napkin rings, my intern Minsu and I would focus on setting a positive intention for the recipient. I even set them outside during a full moon to be cleared and charged.

One month after the launch, as everything seemed to be going along swimmingly, disaster hit. I started hearing back that the one-of-a-kind crystals that I spent care adhering to a silver ring fell apart in transit. I was mortified. Every magazine editor in town was opening up my beautifully handmade birchwood box to see . . . a complete mess.

I didn't know if it was due to the summer heat during delivery, improper packaging, or a cohesion issue. All I knew was that before delivery, I could not even remove the solidly adhered crystals with a set of pliers and brute force, and here they were sliding off and looking awful upon arrival. I experienced swells of sadness, embarrassment, and futility while questioning my entrepreneurial worth. In the depths of it, I cried to my mom and best friend that "maybe I should give up." Their words of encouragement lifted me just enough out of my woe-is-me abyss to reach out to an adhesive expert. Then my brother-in-law called and said, "My work makes adhesives! Let me take them to my lab." If only I hadn't sent them out already to every single relevant shelter magazine under the sun.

The hot sun. The 140-degree-in-an-un-air-conditoned-delivery-truck-that-caused-my-adhesive-to-weaken sun.

This is what I learned: No matter what, in business as in life, there are going to be unforeseen snafus and blindsiding stumbling blocks. You can do your due diligence with preparation for such things (like I did with the numbers, legalities, research, marketing, quality control, SEOs, etc.), but you should always count on the fact that there will be an event that can range from a crisis to a simple disappointment that you never expected. It all comes down to how you handle it. Upon hearing the news of my crystal beauties' disastrous arrivals, did I immediately say to myself, "No big deal! I'm on it!"? Not exactly. I wallowed in capitalist self-doubt and even cried. Hardly the behavior of an experienced and stoic CEO. (Remember that chapter about briefly going to the dark in order to realistically get to more light? This is an important cog in the wheel of self-progress.) Nevertheless, within two days I got back on track. Plunging downward to stop, pause (but not get stuck there), reflect, and regroup enabled me to more solidly focus on going forward, and now the company has grown tremendously.

Tackling a disappointing event in a complete and holistic mind/body/spirit/space manner involved addressing all areas of the whole. The "mind" portion was allowing myself to fully experience any emotion that came with this situation—not squelch it down or move too rapidly to "it's no big deal." If you skip over or suppress this part, it is bound to snowball and erupt later on in a big, messy, misplaced way, like a sudden explosive freak-out at a loved one or an over-the-top road rage flare-up. Forget the "suck it up" mentality. If you need to brood and wallow in your troubles to experience the whole process, do it. (Just don't get stuck here). The "body" is the direct action, and involves formulating a practical plan to get through it. (In this case finding a specific expert to weigh in, getting scientific testing done.) If this situation were happening to your best friend, what would your realistic advice be to get through it? Be your own best friend here, and advise yourself on the necessary steps to the other side. "Spirit" covered the energetic aspects.

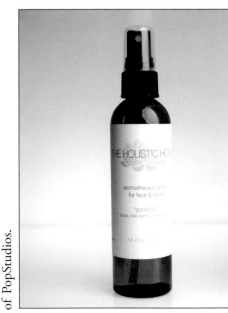

Photos of Holistic Home Company products courtesy of PopStudios.

I sprayed "The Holistic Home Company Good Juju Aromatherapy Spray" throughout my home and work space. This spray contains a powerful trifecta of essential oils of sage, palo santo, and frankincense. Singularly, each one has a strong history through the ages of energetically clearing a space, but together, all three are astounding at releasing negative energy and purifying the spirit.

Dealing with a faulty product was heartbreaking. However, only through failure and hard work could I ever attempt to achieve success and excellence in quality control by ardently striving for improvement. I don't look for perfection in people or things or in my home. That is fruitless and tiring. For me, it's in the full circle arc from moving along "swimmingly" to suddenly sinking and then coming back up for air to go forward in a better way. Perfection is more of the process itself of unabridged improvement by learning from mistakes and aligning *all the parts of you* together as you go. It's the work of your soul.

Here I am, fourteen years from when I was diagnosed with four years to live. In order, I've gone through a change in diagnosis, a switch in career, two moves, got married, had a child, consulted, lectured, and taught regularly, launched a new business, and have written this book throughout it all. I've learned how to holistically tackle the cycles, lessons, mistakes, and successes, which have enabled me to help my clients, and now you, dear reader, to reach your own desired transformations in a more pragmatic and all-inclusive way. By doing the work—clearing out, heeding the cues, decoding the symbolism, aligning, balancing, living with sustainability and intention—as this book has described, you can truly live a life that is richer, healthier, and more meaningful, one that also reinforces your goals and the best you. As you grow and evolve, so should your home, and changes should be made to support your next cycles. Hopefully, maybe now you don't have to wait for life to hit you on the head to make that clear. It can all begin right now, in you and in your home. Your Holistic Home.

Wishing you all things good for your mind, body, spirit, and space.

Acknowledgments

First, I'd like to thank the publishers that "didn't get it" and rejected this number one bestseller and all the people who said it would never happen. All of you strengthened my determination to make this book come true against all odds. And now for the strong and mighty pack that always had my back (and my BFF, who has been planning her book-signing outfit for several years) and those who believed in me from day one:

Thank you to my Big Daddy, Gene S. Benko, who has been an inspiration to me throughout this book and in every minute of my life. My mother, Barbara Benko, whose mantra, "This book will happen!" has cheered me on endlessly, lifted me with every fall and felt all my sorrows and joys deeper than her own. You two are the greatest, most supportive, loving, and selfless parents, and this book is because of you. Thank you to my sister in blood and spirit, Lisa Rodriguez, for being my backbone of support, intuitive medicine woman, and soulful confidante throughout my life. Thank you, Carlos Rodriguez, for all your generosity, positive support, and belief in The Holistic Home Company.

Thank you to my best friend, Andrea Sanders—the greatest unofficial editor—who made me a better writer, who is always an understanding voice of reason, and who fills me with peace, laughter, and balance. Thank you to the dashing and witty Phillip Tyler Alden. Your humor, friendship, iChats, and thank-you cards make my life complete.

Thank you for everything, Leigh and Jim Gardner, Katherine and Mary Benko, Rebecca Tracey, Nichole Thompson Adams, Susan Fisher Plotner, the brilliantly creative Keith Gallic, and my dearest, sweetest Grandma, Helen Kaye, whom I feel with me everyday.

Thank you to Nicole Frail and everyone at Skyhorse/Helios for all your diligent work and professionalism. My deepest gratitude goes to all my clients who opened up their hearts and homes to transformation and inspired me to write this book.

Lastly, I'd like to thank my favorite two. To my hardworking and loving husband, John Ceriello, thank you for letting me pursue this dream, for being my patient and easy-going man, and for being an incredible father to our daughter. And finally, my little nibblet, my shining star, my extraordinary girl, Luchia Skye Ceriello. Never give up on your dreams, work hard, be kind, speak up, and persevere, because you can do anything.

The Holistic Home Index

A

Acupuncture, 64–65
Americana Manhasset, 200–203
Angels, 171
Apartment Therapy, 162
Aromatherapy, 92, 103, 131, 174, 198, 209, 210

B

Bagua
    descriptions of, 43–44
    map, 42, 45, 46
    multiple ways to place, 46
    troubleshooting, 47
Bamboo, 76, 197
Bell, John Stewart, 60
Benko, Barbara, 148, 217
Benko, Gene, 21–24
Brooklyn, 2, 12, 210
Byrne, Lorna, 171

C

Castagna, Frank, 201
Cedarwood, 177
Chakra, 81
Champions For Charity, 202
Chronotherapy, 67
Classroom, 121
Clearing ceremony, 52, 53–55
Closets, 88, 89, 93, 97, 98
Clutter
    and the body, 32–33
    identifying the source, 19
    kids and clutter, 37–38
    mental clutter, 15, 19
    physical clutter, 19, 24, 32
    spiritual clutter, 49–52

Colors, 162–163
Community, 189–190
COMO, Parrot Cay, 204
Consultation
    typical consultation, 9–12
    what to expect, 5
Craigslist, 147, 151
Crystals, 212, 213

D

Dark side, 17
De-cluttering
    de-cluttering your mind, 18–20
    physically de-cluttering, 33–35
Decorating guidelines, 155–157
Design*Sponge, 162
Desk, placement of, 112–115
Doors, 165–166

E

Earth, 67, 68, 70, 72, 80, 164, 187
Electrical Magnetic Fields, 10, 118
Elements, 62, 66–67, 68, 80, 163, 186–187
Emotional Sustainability, 173–176
Eucalyptus, 177

F

Fabrics, 69, 147, 170, 179
Fasano, Susan, 105–108
Fear
    clutter and, 30
    how it shows up, 31–32
    solutions for, 31–32
    types of, 31–32
Feng Shui
    map of, 10, 41–42

misconceptions of, 7
schools of, 39–40
Feng Shui for Dummies, 112
Fire, 66, 68, 69, 80, 163, 186
Firecrackers, 3, 90
Five Elements
    and the body, 66–68
    and the mind, 71
    overview of, 68–69
    reaching goals, 71–72
    spirit of, 79–82
    table of, 68
    theory of, 58, 64, 65
Foliage
    benefits of, 76
    chart of, 76
Foo dogs, 3, 90
Frankincense, 52, 193, 214
Front door
    Bagua placement of, 47
    enhancing the chi of, 8

G

Garden, 186
Green Living, 4
Gua, 41

H

Hall, Carla, 142
Hamptons West, 105
Holistic
    definition of, 4
    excellence, 196, 204–209
    Holistic Home Company, 209–215
Hospital, 197–200
Hulburt, Jenni, 174
Huntington, Benjamin, 42

I

I Ching, 41, 59, 60
Ingebretson, Sue, 193–194
Intention, 142
Interior design, 127, 143–144

J

Johnson, Bea, 181–182
Judge Judy, 22

K

Karan, Donna, 199, 200
Karma, 75, 180–181
Kennedy, David Daniel, 112

L

Lavender, 174–175, 177
Lemon, 92, 93, 103, 174, 177
Lighting, 169–170
Lotus, 184

M

Mantra, 16
Marino, Peter, 200
Medication, 67
Meditation, 16
Merollo, Danielle, 201
Metal, 43, 60, 66, 68, 71, 80, 164,
    187
Mirrors, 31, 103, 114, 119,
    164–165
Moving, 194–195
Myelofibrosis, 1, 2
Myelogenous leukemia, 3

N

NASA, 75, 77
Nature, 56–60, 63, 155
Neat freak, living with a, 36–37
Nostalgia, 27–29

O

Office, 120–121
Organ Clock Theory, 64, 67
Organization, 4, 5, 37, 92

P

Palo santo, 53, 214
Parrot Cay, 204, 208
Plants (benefits of), 75–77
Polycythemia, 3
Position
    bed position, 118–120
    desk position, 120, 121
    stove position, 117–118
Prayer, 16–17
Psychology, 4, 5, 10, 39

R

Red, 3, 61, 68, 69, 71, 162, 186
Rituals, 9, 52, 53, 192, 193
Rosemary, 177

S

Sage
    dried, 54
    essential oil of, 214
Sanders, Andrea, 202
Seasons, 217
Slob, living with a, 36
Soul
    creating a home with, 142
Spirituality
    inviting it into your home,
        171–172
Stairs, 165–166
Sustainability
    emotional sustainability,
        173–176
    physical sustainability, 177–179
    spiritual sustainability, 179–181
Symbolism
    addressing holistically, 90–93
    hidden symbolism, 88–90
    in relationships, 94–95

T

Tao, 60, 77
Textures, 170
Thyme, 177
Toms, 210
Tracey, Rebecca, 64, 217

U

Urban Zen, 199

V

Van Sweden, Oehme, 200

W

Walls, 170–171
Warby Parker, 210
Water
    decorating with, 163–164
    element of, 66, 68, 70, 80,
        163–164, 186–187
    in the garden, 186
    moving or still, 188–189
Wealth
    bagua, 43, 50
    colors of, 43
Weischeit, Regina, 149–152
Windows, 93, 102, 166
Wood
    decorating with, 163
    element of, 66, 68, 70, 80, 163,
        187–188
    wood furniture, 169

Y

Yin and Yang
    lessons of the soul, 137–138
    theory, 127
    throughout the bagua, 138–140
    within yourself, 140–141

Z

Zero Waste Lifestyle, 181–182